VERY EARLY
RECOGNITION OF
CORONARY
HEART DISEASE

VERY EARLY RECOGNITION OF CORONARY HEART DISEASE

Based on a Symposium arranged by the
Cardiothoracic Institute, associated with the
National Heart and Chest Hospitals, and held
at the Royal College of Physicians, London,
on the 4th and 5th May, 1977

Edited by

LAWSON McDONALD M.A., M.D., F.R.C.P., F.A.C.C.
JOHN GOODWIN M.D., F.R.C.P., F.A.C.C.
and
LEON RESNEKOV M.D. (Cape Town), F.R.C.P.

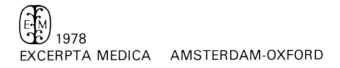 1978
EXCERPTA MEDICA   AMSTERDAM-OXFORD

International Congress Series No. 435
ISBN 0 444 90007 1

Library of Congress Cataloging in Publication Data
Main entry under title:
Very early recognition of coronary heart disease.

Includes indexes.
1. Coronary heart disease--Diagnosis--Congresses. I. McDonald, Lawson. II. Goodwin, John F. III. Resnekov, Leon. IV. Cardiothoracic Institute. V. Royal College of Physicians of London.
RC685.C6V47   616.1'23'075   78-2019
ISBN 0-444-90007-1

Publisher:
Excerpta Medica
305 Keizersgracht
Amsterdam
P.O. Box 1126

Sole Distributors for the USA and Canada:
Elsevier/North-Holland Inc.
52 Vanderbilt Avenue
New York, NY 10017

Printed in The Netherlands by Drukkerij Groen, IJmuiden.

Speakers and chairmen

RAPHAEL BALCON, Dean, Cardiothoracic Institute; Physician, London Chest Hospital, London.

DAVID BLANKENHORN, Professor of Medicine, Head of Cardiology, University of Southern California, Los Angeles, U.S.A.

ROBERT BRUCE, Professor of Medicine, Co-Director, Division of Cardiology, University of Washington, Seattle, Washington, U.S.A.

WALLACE BRIGDEN, Physician, National Heart Hospital and London Hospital; Lecturer, Cardiothoracic Institute, London.

JOHN COLTART Physician, St. Thomas's Hospital, London.

DEREK GIBSON, Physician, Brompton Hospital, London.

JOHN GOODWIN, Professor of Clinical Cardiology, Royal Postgraduate Medical School; Physician, Hammersmith Hospital, London.

PETER HARRIS, Simon Marks Professor of Cardiology, Cardiothoracic Institute; Physician, National Heart Hospital, London.

WALTER HOLLAND, Professor of Clinical Epidemiology and Social Medicine, St. Thomas's Hospital Medical School, London.

DESMOND JULIAN, Professor of Cardiology, University of Newcastle, Newcastle upon Tyne.

BRUCE KOTTKE, Head, Cardiovascular Research Unit, Mayo Clinic, Rochester, Minnesota, U.S.A.

DENNIS KRIKLER, Physician, Hammersmith Hospital and King Edward Memorial Hospital; Lecturer, Royal Postgraduate Medical School, London.

CLIVE LAYTON, Physician, London Chest Hospital.

ATTILIO MASERI, Professor of Cardiology, Clinical Physiology, Laboratory of the National Council for Research, Pisa, Italy.

LAWSON McDONALD, Physician, National Heart Hospital and London Hospital; Lecturer, Cardiothoracic Institute, London.

ANTHONY MITCHELL, Professor of Medicine, University of Nottingham, Nottingham.

BERTRAM PITT, Associate Professor of Medicine, Director, Specialized Center of Research for Ischemic Heart Disease, Johns Hopkins Medical Institutions, Baltimore, Maryland, U.S.A.

LEON RESNEKOV, Professor and Joint Director, Department of Medicine (Cardiology), University of Chicago, Chicago, U.S.A.

P.S. ROBINSON, St. Thomas's Hospital, London.

COLON SCHWARTZ, Head, Department of Atherosclerosis and Thrombosis Research, Cleveland Clinic, Cleveland, Ohio, U.S.A.

JOHN SHILLINGFORD, Professor of Angiocardiology, Royal Postgraduate Medical School; Physician, Hammersmith Hospital, London.

JOAN SLACK, Clinical Scientific Officer, M.R.C. Clinical Genetics Unit, Institute of Child Health; Physician, Hospital for Sick Children, Great Ormond Street, London.

JEREMY SWAN, Director of Cardiology, Cedars-Sinai Medical Center, Los Angeles, California, U.S.A.

Introduction

The views of world authorities on the rapidly growing field of the very early recognition of coronary heart disease were presented at this international meeting. As medical and surgical treatment advances, the importance of identification and treatment before coronary heart disease has become manifest, and of preventing its advance, is increasingly apparent. This symposium was arranged by Dr. Lawson McDonald, Professor John Goodwin and Dr. Leon Resnekov.

The organisers of the symposium wish to express their appreciation to National Westminster Bank for generous financial support which enabled the overseas speakers to travel to the United Kingdom. Thanks to the generosity of the Leeds Castle Foundation it was possible to hold a preliminary scientific meeting for two days of intensive discussions at Leeds Castle. The organisers wish to thank Lord Geoffrey-Lloyd and the Council of the Foundation for all their help. They also thank the Commercial Union Assurance Company for the financial help towards projection costs.

We are most grateful to Miss Irene Oddy who has greatly helped in the preparation of the publication of the proceedings, and to Mrs. Jean Beresford, Miss Hazel Edwards, Mrs. Catherine McLoughlin, and Miss Susan Segar for unfailing secretarial and other assistance.

Lawson McDonald
John Goodwin
Leon Resnekov

Contents

THE CLINICAL CHALLENGE

Lawson McDonald

National Heart Hospital and Cardiothoracic Institute, London

The ability to diagnose the presence of coronary heart disease in individuals who will later manifest it has become of paramount importance. Methods of medical and surgical treatment for the disease steadily improve, and if these are to be most effective the very early recognition of coronary heart disease, preferably before symptoms have occurred, is vital. The high percentage of individuals with coronary heart disease whose first manifestation is sudden death highlights the problem.

Epidemiological studies and the recognition of the presence of risk factors merely make it possible to place the individual in a high-risk category, but the disease will not occur in many such people. Thus more definitive information is needed. If physicians are to avoid the disturbing situation of a patient dying suddenly or sustaining a heart attack within hours of a medical examination, when he or she may have been pronounced fit, an improved diagnostic approach is needed.

In the very early recognition of coronary heart disease it is now apparent that the individual should frequently be examined both at rest and with exercise, using techniques which vary from a thorough clinical examination to sophisticated methods which may be limited to exceptional studies. The changing state of the individual, the reproducibility of any test, and its sensitivity and specificity, are of extreme importance. Recognition should be given to the possibility of summating various tests to enhance prognostic possibilities.

The approach to the individual will certainly include a critical appraisal of clini-cal symptoms and signs: thereafter investigation may be non-invasive or invasive (1). The circulating blood may be studied in vitro for abnormalities of lipid metabolism and glucose-handling, a potential thrombogenic tendency, and hormonal abnormalities. Coronary arteriography precisely indicates occlusive arterial disease and spasm, but may show no apparent abnormality of the vessel wall. Changes in the structure and function of the heart muscle are increasingly useful as indicators of the presence of early coronary heart disease in studies performed at rest and with exercise. Methods include stress testing with recording of the electrocardiogram and other parameters, ventricular angiography, electrophysiological studies which may reveal electrical instability of the heart, including a tendency to block, echocardiography, cardiac imaging with radioactive isotopes, and biochemical inves-tigation.

These and other approaches will be thoroughly reviewed, the position of established methods revalued, and the possibilities of new ones indicated in the ensuing pages.

REFERENCE

(1) McDonald, L. The very early recognition of coronary heart disease. In: Progress in Cardiology (Yu, P.N. & Goodwin, J.F., Eds.). Philadelphia, Lea and Febiger, to be published.

THE VERY EARLY RECOGNITION OF CORONARY HEART DISEASE - EPIDEMIOLOGY OF RISK FACTORS
IN EARLY LIFE

Walter Holland

St. Thomas's Hospital Medical School, London

Over the last 30 years there has been an increasing volume of literature on the risk
factors associated with coronary artery disease - we do not intend to describe this
here as much of it is well known. Following recognition of these risk factors there
have been many attempts to reverse the progress of the disease by means of intervention in adults but few of these attempts have had a marked effect so it seems
likely that primary prevention in childhood would be more effective if the risk factors can be shown to be present.

Many of the papers presented at this symposium consider the recognition of the disease in terms of symptoms and functional changes. A number of investigations have
already been undertaken to discover if the risk can be altered for individuals with
detected functional changes, for example by treatment to reduce blood pressure levels.
However none of the controlled trials on people with mild to moderate hypertension
identified by screening, have shown any benefit in terms of reduction in mortality
from coronary artery disease. And, despite widespread belief that level of blood
cholesterol is related to incidence of the disease in later life, trials of reduction
in cholesterol intake have been unsuccessful. Attempts to change people's behaviour
by, for example, encouraging them to take more exercise, have been ineffective.

Such investigations show that attempts should be made to alter the incidence of coronary artery disease by detection and measurement of risk factors present in children
and subsequent reduction or removal of these factors.

A number of studies we have undertaken to measure the risk factors in children will
be described here with some ideas about how they may be altered at an early age.

In 1976 Kuller (1) stated that "if coronary atherosclerosis with subsequent coronary
artery stenosis is accepted as the underlying determinant of disease, then several
questions must be pursued to improve our understanding of the disease:
1. What is the age of onset of coronary atherosclerosis and the determinants of the
    initial disease process?
2. What is the rate of progression of coronary atherosclerosis from fatty streaks to
    fibrous plaques to complicated lesions and then to coronary artery stenosis?
3. Is there a critical degree of coronary artery stenosis required for the appear-
    ance of clinical disease?"
To answer at least the first question epidemiological studies have identified a number of risk factors associated with the development and progression of coronary artery disease. Cigarette smoking, level of blood pressure, weight and cholesterol and
fat intake and level of activity are commonly implicated. Some studies have also
been concerned with psycho-social and personality factors.

Results from the following studies reveal some important findings with implications
for preventive action in the future.

Blood Pressure
It has been suggested that higher blood pressure in young adulthood leads to a faster
rate of increase with age but it may be simply that high levels in young adulthood

are followed by higher levels with advancing age. In either case there does appear
to be a tracking effect with age but what determines the track for an individual is
as yet unknown.

There is considerable evidence that hereditary factors play an important role; a
number of studies have examined the relationship between blood pressures of parents
and children and of children and their siblings. However, as Johnson and colleagues
(2) have pointed out, the interaction of environmental factors such as social class
or family background on genetically susceptible people is also important in determining the incidence of disease whatever the hereditary factors. Miall, Bell and Lovell
(3) have shown that physical characteristics such as body build and weight also influence the blood pressures of young adults.

There have been a number of studies of familial aggregation of blood pressure but
only in populations aged 15 and older until Kass in 1971 (4) studied families with
children aged 2 - 14. However because his group was taken from families where the
mother had been examined for bacteriuria during pregnancy the families were highly
selected. A number of other similar studies have now been done (5, 6, 7, 8) and we
will describe here one by Beresford and Holland in 1973 (5).

The sample of 568 families was drawn from families who had a child born between 1
July 1963 and 30 June 1965. Each family was visited once in 1970 or 1971 when the
children were six or seven years old: blood pressure measurements were taken twice
for each family member. It was found that although systolic pressure of the child
was associated with that of both father and mother, the most important factor influencing the child's blood pressure was his or her own weight. Social class also
appeared to be slightly associated with blood pressure but no other environmental
factors investigated seemed to influence it. Thus weight, a factor associated with
blood pressure in adults is already of importance in childhood.

A further study in Kent (Rona, R., unpublished data) has shown that children who have
higher blood pressure levels than their peers in one year tend to have the same in
the following year (Figure 1). This study indicates a tracking effect of blood pressure levels.

Plasma Sugar and Serum Cholesterol
In several studies in adults a weak but significant association has been found between blood pressure and plasma sugar measured after an oral challenge (Epstein, F.H.:
Obesity: hyperglycemia and hypertension. Sixth World Congress of Cardiology, London,
1970. Unpublished data) (9 - 13). This relationship was found to be much stronger
in schoolchildren aged 9 - 12 by Florey and colleagues (14) who also found that plasma sugar in boys was even more closely associated with blood pressure than was weight.
They showed that boys with plasma sugar levels above 7 mmol/l tended to have systolic
blood pressures about 10 mm Hg higher than those with plasma sugar or levels below 5
mmol/l independently of weight, and in girls a similar but slightly smaller difference was found.

Florey and colleagues also found that serum cholesterol was associated with blood
pressure independently of weight and blood sugar in boys but not in girls. This
difference between the sexes was also found in studies of white American adults (13),
in an adult population in Chicago (9) and in French civil servants (12). Similar
analyses of data from a rural Jamaican population, in which myocardial infarction is
rare, showed no association between blood pressure and one hour blood sugar or serum
cholesterol (15). These findings suggest that in countries where clinical coronary
heart disease is common in middle aged men there is an association between the three
major risk factors for the disease and this association is detectable in childhood.

Obesity
It has been apparent for some time that obesity is related to a number of diseases in

later life including hypertension and coronary artery disease. Some studies have suggested that overweight children become overweight adults although evidence for this is not conclusive.

It is recognised that weight alone is a poor measure of obesity and Newens and Goldstein (16) have criticised the assumption that a given centile of weight indicates the same degree of relative adiposity for children of the same age but different height. They also showed that the more simple approach of analysing weight by height regardless of age is inaccurate.

The National Study of Health and Growth (17) has been running since 1972: it is a system of yearly growth surveillance of over 10,000 primary school-children in 28 employment exchange areas of England and Scotland. The data of weight and height collected in this survey have enabled construction of standards of weight by height and age. In the form of 'confidence contours' these standards of weight by height and age could be used to screen for obesity (18).

Figure 2 illustrates contours of weight by height and age from data collected in 1972. It shows the 97 and 80 per cent contours enclosing those percentages for a particular age group. Figure 3 shows a practical use of this method. It shows the confidence contours derived from the data for English seven year old boys with Scottish seven year old boys plotted on it. The average height, weight and regression of weight on height of the English boys show the relative position of the Scottish boys: half of the boys in the sample were under the regression line and half were over showing that Scottish and English boys are of similar build in this particular example. Figure 4 shows the relationship between weight and height contours for successive years.

These confidence contours could be used as a method of assessing overweight for height by age and sex but further work is needed to assess their validity and practicality for short term follow-up of overweight in individual children. If overweight - as defined by using such contours - is a good predictor of obesity then the technique could be used to screen for overweight children and possibly combine dietary education with regular blood pressure checks.

Smoking
For several years we have been involved in studies of smoking in school-children in Kent and Derbyshire (19 - 24). It has been shown that there are certain factors associated with children's smoking. These are: (i) having parents who smoke - this appears to be sex-related, that is boys are more likely to smoke if their fathers smoke and girls are more likely to smoke if their mothers smoke (23); (ii) having siblings who smoke - this factor does not appear to be sex-related (24); (iii) having friends inside and outside school who smoke; (iv) academic ability, children who felt they were doing well at school and whose head teachers ranked them as good academically (without knowledge of their smoking) were less likely to be smokers (23); (v) truancy children who play truant are more likely to be smokers (24); (vi) type of school - secondary school children attending secondary modern schools are more likely to smoke than those attending comprehensive or grammar schools (22, 25, 26) (but this may be because of selection for schools and social class differences); (vii) children's attitude to their own health.

In view of the importance of smoking in the development of coronary artery disease it is obvious that there must be early intervention to prevent children from taking up smoking. It may be possible to influence some of the factors associated with smoking. In particular this applies to parents and the peer group (Table I). Teachers' attitudes in school could also be influenced and altering children's own attitudes by increasing their awareness of the immediate respiratory effects of smoking, in relation to general fitness, and also their knowledge of smoking related diseases, such

TABLE 1

	FACTORS INFLUENCING CHILDREN'S SMOKING		INTERVENTION FOR REDUCTION OF CHILDREN'S SMOKING
FAMILY and FRIENDS	Parents		Education of pregnant mothers
	Siblings	)	
	Friends	))	Peer group influence
	Type of school		Attitudes of teachers and peer group
PERSONAL FACTORS	Academic ability	)	
	Truancy	)))	All these are inter-related and related to type of school and all are difficult to change
	Rebelliousness (anticipation of adulthood)	))	
	Children's attitudes towards health		Knowledge of smoking - related diseases, both acute/chronic

as coronary artery disease and lung cancer, is important.

It is hoped that further research into smoking habits of school-children will include a study to discover if a particular health education programme is effective in altering children's smoking habits.

Conclusion
Since there appears to be a tracking effect of blood pressure with age, whereby an individual who has a higher blood pressure at one age is likely to have high blood pressure at a second age, it should be possible to identify children with high blood pressure and keep them under surveillance. Alternatively if one or both parents have high blood pressure then the children should be examined and kept under surveillance if necessary. Again since weight and blood pressure have been shown to be related in children those who are overweight could be identified and their blood pressure kept under surveillance.

In the context of the relationship between blood pressure and plasma sugar which is independent of weight the preventive measure of weight reduction is not relevant. The finding of raised plasma sugar level associated with raised blood pressure may simply be an artefact of the physical examination: in more nervous children secretion of catecholamines could raise both blood pressure and plasma sugar levels. If this is not so both short and long term experiments are needed in order to discover whether the plasma sugar levels determine blood pressure or vice versa. If it can be confirmed that reduction of plasma sugar or response to an oral glucose challenge is followed by a reduction in blood pressure appropriate preventive action - probably dietary - can be considered.

As we know that weight is a risk factor associated with coronary artery disease and if we can decide what constitutes overweight in children then attempts must be made to reduce their weight to prevent them becoming overweight adults. If there is a consequent reduction in blood pressure this hopefully will be associated with a reduction in the incidence of coronary artery disease.

A number of the risk factors associated with children taking up smoking have been established and it is possible that some of these may be influenced but as yet we are unaware how children may be discouraged from taking up the habit.

Now we know the risk factors associated with coronary artery disease further help is required from social scientists and health educationalists to make use of current methods of intervention and develop new ones in order to reduce the incidence of coronary artery disease by primary prevention.

REFERENCES

(1) Kuller, L.H. (1976): Amer. J. Epidem., 104 (4), 425.
(2) Johnson, B.C., Epstein, F.H. and Kjelsberg, M.O. (1965): J. Chron. Dis., 18, 147.
(3) Miall, W.E., Bell, R.A. and Lovell, H.G. (1968): Brit. J. Prev. Soc. Med., 22, 73.
(4) Zinner, S.H., Levy, P.S. and Kass, E.H. (1971): New Engl. J. Med., 284, 401.
(5) Beresford, S.A.A. and Holland, W.W. (1973): Proc. Roy. Soc. Med., 66, 10.
(6) Kass, E.H., Zinner, S.H. and Margolius, H.S. et al. (1975): In: Paul O., ed. Epidemiology and Control of Hypertension, Stratton Intercontinental Medical Books, New York, p. 359.
(7) Klein, B.E., Hennekens, C.H. and Jesse, M.J. et al. (1975): In: Paul O., ed. Epidemiology and Control of Hypertension, Stratton Intercontinental Medical Books, New York, p. 387.
(8) Beaglehole, R., Salmond, C.E. and Prior, I.A.M. (1975): In: Paul O., ed.

Epidemiology and Control of Hypertension, Stratton Intercontinental Medical Books, New York, p. 407.

(9) Stamler, J., Rhomberg, P. and Schoenberger, J.A. et al. (1975): J. Chron. Dis., 28, 527.

(10) Stamler, J., Stamler, R. and Rhomberg, P. et al. (1975): J. Chron. Dis., 28, 499.

(11) Jarrett, J. and Keen, H. (1975): In: Complications of Diabetes, ed. Keen H. and Jarrett, J., Arnold, London, p. 179.

(12) Eschwege, E., Valleron, A.J. and Rosselin, G.E. et al. (1975): In: Diabetes Epidemiology in Europe, eds. Cutsche, H. and Holler, H.D., George Thieme, Stuttgart, p. 120.

(13) Florey, C. du V. and Acheson, R.M. (1969): Vital and Health Stats. PHS Pub. No. 1000 Ser. 11, No. 34, Washington D.C.

(14) Florey, C. du V., Uppal, S. and Lowy, C. (1976): Brit. Med. J., 1, 1368.

(15) Florey, C. du V., McDonald H., McDonald, J. and Miall, W.E. (1972): Int. J. Epid., 1, 157.

(16) Newens, E.M. and Goldstein, H. (1972): Brit. J. Prev. Soc. Med., 26, 33.

(17) Irwig, L.M. (1976): Int. J. Epid., 5, 57.

(18) Rona, R. and Altman, D.G. (1977): National Study of Health and Growth: Standards of attained height, weight and triceps skinfold in English children for 5 - 11 years old. Annals of Human Biology (submitted for publication).

(19) Holland, W.W. and Elliott, A. (1968): Lancet, 1, 41.

(20) Bland, J.M. and Bewley, B.R. (1975): Brit. J. Prev. Soc. Med., 29, 262.

(21) Bland, J.M., Bewley, B.R., Banks, M.H. and Pollard, V. (1975): Health Education Journal, 34, 71.

(22) Bewley, B.R. and Bland, J.M. (1976): Preventive Medicine, 5, 63.

(23) Bewley, B.R. and Bland, J.M. (1977): Academic Performance and Social Factors related to cigarette smoking by school-children. Brit. J. Prev. Soc. Med. (in press).

(24) Banks, M.H., Bewley, B.R. and Bland, J.M. et al. (1977): A long-term study of smoking by secondary school-children (submitted 1977).

(25) Holland, W.W., Halil, T., Bennett, A.E. and Elliott, A. (1969): Millbank Memorial Quarterly, XLVII, No. 3 (Part 2), 215.

(26) Holland, W.W., Halil, T., Bennett, A.E. and Elliott, A. (1969): Brit. Med. J., 2, 205.

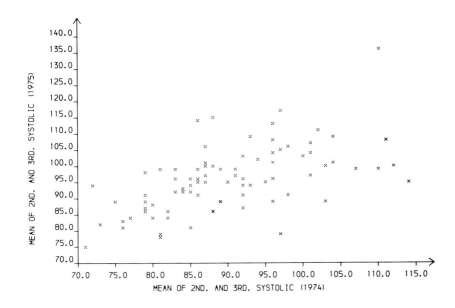

FIG. 1   The year to year association of blood pressure levels in children.

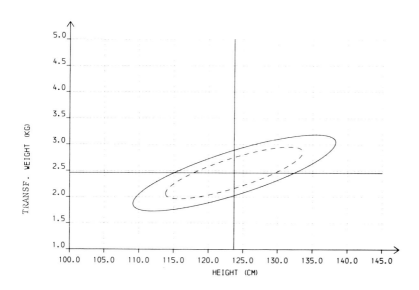

FIG. 2   97 and 80 per cent contours of weight by height for seven year old boys.
Vertical axis gives Transformed Weight = log$_e$ (weight in Kg-12).

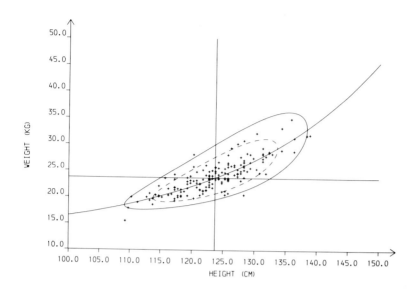

FIG. 3   Contours derived from data from English seven year old boys with data from
          Scottish seven year old boys plotted on it.

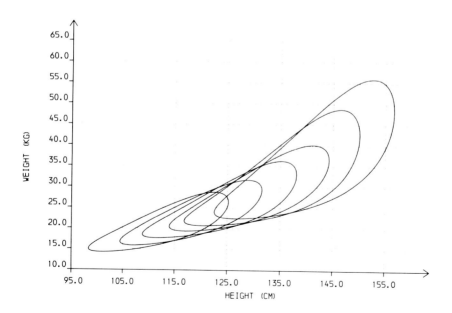

FIG. 4   The 97 per cent weight and height contours for boys for six yearly age-
          groups (5+ - 10+).

10

EARLY METABOLIC PREDICTION IN ADULTS

Joan Slack

Institute of Child Health and Hospital for Sick Children, Great Ormond Street, London

There is a great deal of evidence in the literature for the well known risk factors as predictors of coronary heart disease. This paper aims to compare the predictive value of some of the risk factors, to use the published data to examine the accuracy with which prediction of impending coronary death can be made and to examine the certainty with which those at exceptionally high risk can be detected in the population.

Table 1 shows the magnitude of 2 inescapable risk factors, sex and age. The Registrar General's Statistics for England and Wales (1) show that in 1972 the coronary mortality rate for men between 35 and 44 was 546/million and for women was 80. Between 45 and 64 the coronary mortality rate for men had increased to 6,022/million and for women to 1,627. Thus for men of 40 the increased risk over women of the same age is 6.8 fold and at 60 the increase for males is somewhat less at 3.7 fold. Turning to age as a risk factor, the same figures indicate that the 20 years between 40 and 60 increases the coronary mortality rate for men 11 fold and for women the same advance in age produces a 20 fold increase in risk. If age and sex alone are used to predict coronary death in men and women between 45 and 49 over the subsequent 10 years the Registrar General's Statistics for England and Wales would suggest that if risks remained at the 1972 level 3.2 per cent of the men would die from acute myocardial infarction in the next 10 years and 0.6 per cent of the women.

What improvement can be made on this prediction? The search to improve the prediction of early coronary death has been prodigious and widesweeping; from dietary fibres (8) and soft water (9) through the stresses of public speaking (10) or being a Member of Parliament (11) and more recently to the serum triglyceride levels (12) and the processes of autoimmune disease (13). None of these proposed risk factors has been tested so thoroughly as the more conventional risk factors of blood pressure, serum cholesterol levels or smoking habits and so their predictive strength cannot be compared. I will therefore confine my evaluation to the last three.

The National Pooling Project reported by Stamler and his colleagues in 1970 (2) used several studies to investigate the effects in men of smoking habits, blood pressure and serum cholesterol levels on coronary mortality rates. The Framingham study contributed about one third of the total number of about 7,500 men between 30 and 59 years of age. Figure 1 shows the distribution of diastolic blood pressure of the men entering the study and the coronary mortality rate expressed as a percentage in the subsequent 10 years increasing with increased diastolic pressure. The coronary mortality rate in the whole population was 3.5 per cent, similar to the men in this country. 6.5 per cent of the men had diastolic blood pressure over 105 mm.Hg on entering the study and their coronary mortality rate was 8.9 per cent a 2.5 fold increase over the risk in the population as a whole and a 3 fold increase over those whose blood pressure was less than 75 mm.Hg at the start of the study.

Figure 2 shows the coronary mortality rate associated with serum cholesterol levels in the same study. Serum cholesterol levels were distributed similarly in this population to a population we are studying in N.W. London (3) and the coronary mortality

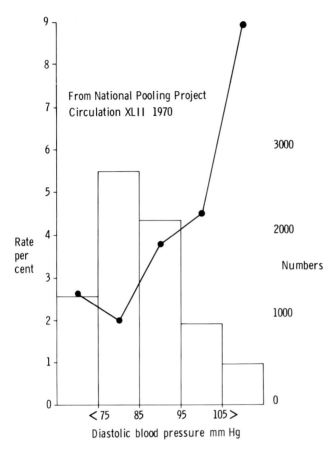

FIG. 1   Distribution of diastolic blood pressure in men aged 30 - 59 and age adjusted coronary mortality rate in subsequent 10 years.

TABLE 1

CORONARY MORTALITY RATES / MILLION.			
REGISTRAR GENERAL 1972		CATEGORY 410.	
	MEN	WOMEN	INCREASE
AGE 40	546	80	X 6.8
AGE 60	6,022	1,627	X 3.7
INCREASE	X 11.0	X 20.3	

rate in the whole population was 3.3 per cent in the subsequent 10 years. 8.5 per cent of the population had serum cholesterol in excess of 300 mg/100 ml at the start of the study and their risk of coronary death in the next 10 years was 5.8 per cent a risk which was 1.76 times the risk in the population as a whole and 2.4 times the risk of those whose serum cholesterol was less than 175 mg/100 ml. A similar order of risk was found in association with smoking more than 20 cigarettes a day. In the population studied 15.4 per cent were smoking more than 20 a day and their risk was 5.9 per cent compared with 3.4 per cent in the population as a whole, or 2.2 per cent among those who had never smoked.

These findings are summarized in Table 2. The three risk factors have been listed in order of their apparent predictive power, an important factor is the proportion of the population detected at each arbitrary cut-off point. For example a diastolic blood pressure of 105 mm.Hg is associated with the highest risk, but this was found in only 6.5 per cent of the population. Serum cholesterol in excess of 300 mg/100 ml was found in 8.5 per cent of the population and at this level cholesterol appears to be the weaker predictor of coronary death. It is not possible from the data provided to estimate the risk of serum cholesterol in excess of the 6.5 percentile and so compares it directly with diastolic blood pressure over 105 mm.Hg.

Finally the data from the Pooling Project shows the coronary mortality among men with a combination of moderate elevation of the three risk factors taking diastolic blood pressure greater than 90 mm.Hg, serum cholesterol greater than 250 mg/100 ml and any cigarette smoking as risk factors they showed that even at these modest levels smoking associated with either hypertension or hypercholesterolaemia increases the risk of coronary death by a factor of 1.7 while the combination of all three increases the risk by more than 2 fold.

How accurate are the predictions from these three risk factors? Taking the highest risk factor, Diastolic Blood Pressure over 105 mm.Hg the findings of The National Pooling Project would suggest that of 1,000 men screened 65 would be found to be at risk with an 8.9 per cent chance of coronary death in the next 10 years and six of these men would be expected to die from coronary heart disease while 59 would survive. Meanwhile 54 coronary deaths would be expected among the remaining 935 of the population not considered at this high risk.

Serum cholesterol is even less helpful for accurate prediction. Out of 1,000 men screened 170 would be expected to have cholesterol levels greater than 275 mg/100 ml and 9 would be expected to die from coronary heart disease in the next 10 years, while 41 deaths would be expected among the remaining 830. This order of accuracy in prediction is not very helpful and many people would think that the anxieties and insurance problems aroused by identifying men with these orders of risk outweigh the usefulness of the predictions. The National Pooling Project does not relate cholesterol levels to the age of the men entering the study and we have found in a recent study of 1,500 men and women working in N.W. London that age has a very significant effect upon serum cholesterol levels.

Figure 3 shows the curvilinear relationship between serum cholesterol concentration and age.

A recent report from the Royal College of Physicians and the British Cardiac Society (7) recommended that men between 30-50 should be specially selected for treatment for prevention of coronary heart disease. The shaded block shows the implications of this recommendation. At 30 years of age, 5 per cent of the population would be included at the lower limit but at the upper limit less than 2 per cent of the population would be eligible for treatment. At 50, the recommended lower limit is less than 1 standard deviation above the mean so that as many as 21 per cent of the male population would be recommended for treatment. At 20 which is perhaps a more promi-

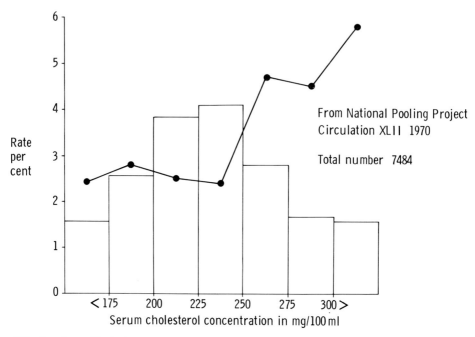

FIG. 2 Age adjusted coronary mortality rate by serum cholesterol concentration in subsequent 10 years.

TABLE 2

INCREASED RISK OF CORONARY DEATH IN MEN AGED 30-59 IN SUBSEQUENT 10 YEARS. STAMLER et al., Circulation, 1970.			
Risk Factor	% Risk of Coronary death	Increase	% Population Affected
Diastolic BP > 105 mm Hg	8.9	x 2.5	6.5
Smoking > 20 cigs./day	5.9	x 1.7	15.4
Serum Cholesterol > 300 mg/100 ml	5.8	x 1.8	8.5
Smoking any cigs. + Cholesterol > 250 mg/100 ml or Diastolic BP > 90 mm Hg	5.5	x 1.7	24.4
Smoking any cigs. + Cholesterol > 250 mg/100 ml + Diastolic BP > 90 mm Hg	7.1	x 2.2	8.1

14

sing time to try to prevent elevation of serum cholesterol no recommendation was made but if it applied the lower limit would identify less than 1 per cent of the population. The recommendation of arbitrary limits as risk factors without regard to their distribution or variations in the population could result in failure to treat the people who should be treated or alternatively could start an overwhelming community health programme whose feasibility must be in some doubt.

Are there any better predictors for early coronary death? While diastolic blood pressure, serum cholesterol and smoking cigarettes is associated with a $2\frac{1}{2}$ to 2 fold increase of early coronary death, the history of coronary death in a first degree relative may carry a somewhat stronger prediction.

Table 3 shows the result of a family study of survivors of myocardial infarction in which Slack and Evans (4) found that for the male relatives of female patients who had their first infarction under 65 years of age there was a 6 fold increase in risk of coronary death before 55, for their female relatives there was a 7 fold increase. For the young male relatives of male patients under 55 there was a 5 fold increase and for their female relatives there was an increased risk in the order of $2\frac{1}{2}$ fold but the numbers for this group were not statistically significant.

If this order of risk was upheld by a prospective study the predictive value of early coronary death in a first degree relative would be stronger than the conventional cut off point for cholesterol or diastolic blood pressure as risk factors. But the family history can be more useful than that, it can alert the physician to the possibility of the highest risk of all, that of dominantly inherited Familial Hypercholesterolaemia. The prediction of death in early adult life in people who inherit 2 mutant genes for this condition is about 100 per cent. For the male heterozygotes the risk of first attack of ischaemic heart disease before the age of 50 is 50 per cent and the risk of death before 60 is also 50 per cent (5). This prediction is so high that identification of these individuals at risk seems to be a compelling need if prevention is to be attempted.

The homozygote frequency in the population is very rare. Only 7 are known in this country, and from this the heterozygote frequency, calculated by the Hardy Weinberg equation is of the order of 1 in 500.

How can the heterozygote be identified in the general population? Affected adults have hypercholesterolaemia, may have tendinous xanthomata, and they may have other affected first degree relatives, but identification of the heterozygote by serum cholesterol levels alone is very difficult. Among those whose cholesterol is elevated above the 95 centile 1 in 25 would be expected to be hypercholesterolaemic because they were heterozygous for Familial Hypercholesterolaemia. Among survivors of myocardial infarction we found 1 in 4 had cholesterol elevated more than 2 standard deviations above the expected level (6) and of these 1 in 4, or 1 in 16 of all the survivors of myocardial infarction, were likely to be heterozygotes for Familial Hypercholesterolaemia and of course 1 in 2 of the children of these heterozygotes will be affected with the mutant gene for Familial Hypercholesterolaemia.

But even among the children of heterozygotes for Familial Hypercholesterolaemia where 1 in 2 will be affected there is some problem in diagnosis. Figure 4 shows the distribution of cholesterol levels in children of heterozygotes referred for treatment to Great Ormond Street Children's Hospital. Log transformation has been used to minimize the skewed distribution most apparent in the upper mode and a maximum likelihood technique has been used to find the best fit. The dotted lines show that the most likely distribution of serum cholesterol levels was bimodal and it seems likely that the upper mode is produced by the heterozygotes. The 2 modes are not equal in size because some children of heterozygotes are screened at other centres and if they are normal are never referred to the hospital.

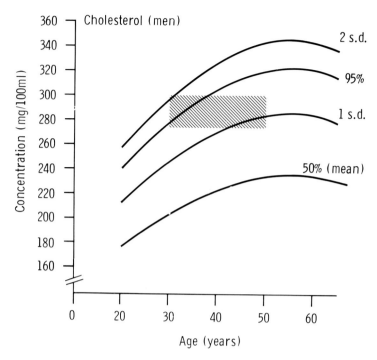

FIG. 3   Age specific values for serum cholesterol in white men at 1 standard deviation above the mean, at 95th centile and at 2 standard deviations above
the mean. Shaded areas indicate definitions of hyperlipidaemia in
"Prevention of Coronary Heart Disease".

TABLE 3

INCREASED RISK OF EARLY CORONARY DEATH IN FIRST DEGREE RELATIVES OF INDEX PATIENTS. SLACK AND EVANS 1966.	
MALE PATIENTS under 55	
MALE RELS. under 55	5.61 ***
FEMALE RELS. under 65	2.75
FEMALE PATIENTS under 65	
MALE RELS. under 55	6.44 ***
FEMALE RELS. under 65	6.92 ***

The mean serum cholesterol of the heterozygotes was 8.9 mmol/l (343 mg/100 ml) and that of the unaffected children was 4.9 mmol/l (188 mg/100 ml). The 2 curves when adjusted to be of equal size intersect at 6.77 mmol/l (261 mg/100 ml). The proportion of children who have values greater than 6.77 is 5 per cent and the proportion of heterozygotes with values less than 6.77 is 3.5 per cent. If the intercept, 6.77 mmol/l, is used to identify heterozygotes in this highly selected population there is liable to be a misdiagnosis in 4.25 per cent of the population at risk.

The probability of making a correct diagnosis of FH among the children of heterozygotes at different levels of serum cholesterol are shown in Figure 5. The probability of being affected if serum cholesterol is 232 or 6 mmol/l is 0.87 while the probability that the child is a heterozygote for Familial Hypercholesterolaemia at a cholesterol level of 290 or 7.5 mmol/l is 0.98. If the same levels in children in the general population are considered the probabilities of the child being affected are very much less and are shown in Figure 6. The probability of a child in the general population with a cholesterol level of 6 mmol/l or 231 mg/100 ml is 0.013 and even at 7.5 mmol or 290 mg/100 ml the probability of correct diagnosis of FH is only 0.10. Indiscriminate population screening then for Familial Hypercholesterolaemia, even in children is likely to be inaccurate until a specific test for heterozygotes is found.

How can we best detect children at high risk for FH? The use of the Family History may be a good compromise. First degree relatives of young patients with ischaemic heart disease with hypercholesterolaemia have a 1 in 8 chance of Familial Hypercholesterolaemia. The probability of correct diagnosis in the children is shown on Figure 7. It is not perfect but it is a considerable improvement on indiscriminate screening of the population, and the risk of early coronary death in the males identified by this selective screening is high. Perhaps this is a way we could identify early those in whom the risks of early coronary death are so high that they must be taken seriously.

In summary, the evidence would suggest that the predictions of coronary heart disease in the population have so far proved quite unsatisfactory and that we should now turn our attention towards selective screening of those who are at specially high risk.

REFERENCES

(1) Registrar General. Statistical Review of England and Wales, Part I, Tables Medical. London. H.M.S.O., 1972.
(2) Stamler, J., Beard, R.R., Connor, W.E., de Wolfe, V.G., Stokes, J. and Willis, P.W. (1970): Circulation, 42, A55.
(3) Slack, J., Noble, N., Meade, T.W. and North, W.R.S. Submitted for publication Brit. Med. J., 1977.
(4) Slack, J. and Evans, K.A. (1966): J. Med. Genet., 3, 239.
(5) Slack, J. (1969): Lancet, 2, 1380.
(6) Patterson, D. and Slack, J. (1972): Lancet, 1, 393.
(7) Prevention of coronary heart disease. Report of a joint working party of the Royal College of Physicians of London and the British Cardiac Society, 1976. J. R. Coll. Physicians Lond., 10, 213.

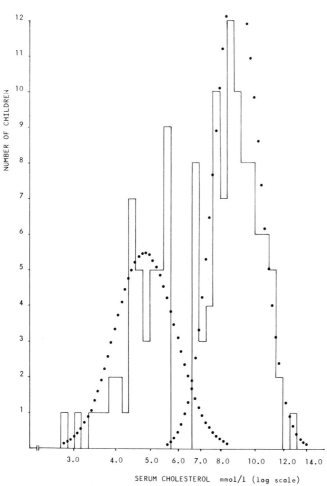

FIG. 4   Distribution of $\log_{10}$ serum cholesterol concentration in children (3 - 16 yrs.) of heterozygotes for Familial Hypercholesterolaemia with maximum likelihood distribution shown...

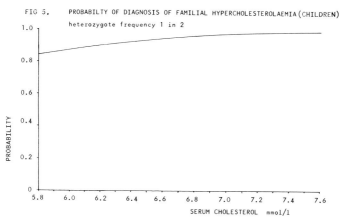

FIG. 5   Probability of diagnosis of Familial Hypercholesterolaemia in children. Heterozygote frequency 1 in 2.

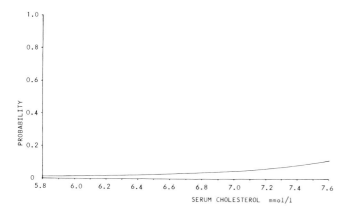

FIG. 6 Probability of diagnosis of Familial Hypercholesterolaemia in children.
Heterozygote frequency 1 in 500.

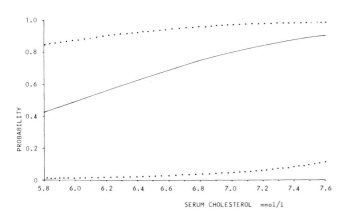

FIG. 7 Probability of diagnosis of Familial Hypercholesterolaemia in children.
Heterozygote frequency 1 in 8.

THE EARLY DETECTION OF THROMBOSIS

Anthony Mitchell

University of Nottingham, Nottingham

The circulating blood is the only part of the cardio-vascular system which can be easily, safely and repetitively biopsied. Whether the study of blood samples will be of value in the early detection of coronary disease depends on a series of unresolved equations involving the inter-relationship of heart muscle disease and coronary artery abnormalities. If Rokitansky's (1) view is correct and thrombosis arises because of an abnormality or 'crasis' in the blood, and that the thrombi give rise to atheromatous plaques, then before these plaques and thrombi have signified their presence by producing sudden death or heart muscle necrosis, we should have been able to detect the abnormality in the blood. If, on the other hand, one accepts Virchow's (2) view that arterial wall disease is not produced by thrombosis, but that artery wall plaques stimulate the passing blood to form thrombi, then our chance of finding a blood abnormality depends on the nature of the local message by which the plaques inform the blood of their existence. If the message is a physical one (turbulent flow, stagnant flow, vortices, etc.) then no discernible change in the general circulating blood would be expected, whereas a chemical message affecting cell or clotting factor activity might well modify the whole of the circulating blood as each round of the circulation brings part of it past the messenger site. Finally, if Spain and Bradess (3) and Baroldi et al. (4) are correct and "heart attacks" are due to the development, in some as-yet mysterious way, of heart muscle necrosis, which in its turn stimulates coronary thrombus formation, then no detectable blood abnormality need antedate the clinical episode since the role of the arteries and their contained blood is secondary and passive.

Two other dilemmas confront the searcher for Rokitansky's crasis; first, the clinical and pathological evidence shows that arterial thrombosis is not an unremitting, continuing process, but rather one of episodes of activity, interspersed with quiescent periods. If there is a "crasis" how can the investigator be sure that he is not carrying out his tests when there is nothing to find? Second, how can the investigator focus down on those individuals who are most likely to show the supposed abnormality? If he embarks on a prospective survey of individuals who are healthy then very large numbers will need to be tested and followed for many years, so that the few who develop clinical evidence of ischaemic heart disease can be detected and their test results can be compared with those who do not. Such an exercise thus involves the collection of a large amount of information, only a fraction of which will bear directly on the problem. Alternatively, the investigator may choose to study individuals who have already revealed themselves to him as being at risk by having had a heart attack. As soon as he concentrates on them he is losing one crucial group - the individuals who do not survive to enter, still less to leave, the unit in which he is based. Moreover, if he studies his patients early in their admission he will be in danger of confusing the consequences of the area of cardiac necrosis (such as altered white cell and platelet counts and behaviour and elevated fibrinogen levels) with its cause. He must therefore wait until the acute episode has resolved, before drawing conclusions about the value of his particular test-system.

Failure on the part of investigators to remember these problems and to document their way of resolving them, has led to the confused and unsatisfactory situation in which we currently find ourselves. We must realise that until we know why flowing liquid blood is able to turn into the solid tissue which we know as a thrombus, we are groping in the dark. In the bone-marrow, the progenitors of the platelets and polymorphonuclear leucocytes which we find in thrombi, adhere to each other to form a solid structure. What property is conferred on them as they mature and are discharged into the moving circulation which makes them non-adherent until they are stimulated? Are they equipped with an "anti-glue" as they leave the marrow, so that thrombosis is the result of a reduced "anti-glue" effect, or is thrombosis due to the evolution of a "glue" which overcomes their natural non-adherence. Searching in the blood for the appearance of a "glue" is potentially easier than hunting for the disappearance of an "anti-glue".

The search for markers of thrombosis

An arterial thrombus is made up of platelets, polymorphonuclear leucocytes and some red cells, held in a fibrin mesh. Most investigators have therefore concentrated on platelet behaviour and on tests of the activity of the fibrin forming (clotting) and fibrin-removing (fibrinolytic) systems. None of the studies so far performed has resolved the basic question - namely, does a detectable blood abnormality antedate and predict the development of clinical coronary disease. However, it is of interest to set out what has been done, to point up the needs for the future.

(a) Blood clotting tests. Because the commonest form of blood-solidification with which we are all familiar is blood clotting, the first half of this century saw an intensive search for clotting-factor differences between normal subjects and various groups (5, 6). Unhappily the majority of these groups were ones that do not allow us to separate the effects of ischaemic heart disease from its possible causes, or were ones in which high-risk groups were compared with low-risk groups but in which the actual predictive value of the groups in terms of eventual clinical events was not put to the test. An early example of the latter, epidemiologically-orientated study was the detailed comparison of blood coagulation mechanisms in white and Bantu men with and without coronary disease (7). This was a study at a given point in time so it was not possible to watch some of the normal subjects develop overt disease and then to scrutinise their preceding clotting factor activity. In any event, there was wide scatter and overlap of individual results, so no predictive value seemed likely to emerge from any specific test. Of much greater interest is the longitudinal epidemiological approach pioneered by Meade and his colleagues (8, 9), in which a large scale prospective study of the link between clotting factors on entry and the subsequent development of vascular disease is under way. As with other major prospective studies, such as Framingham, Tecumseh and the Coronary Drug Project, many years will elapse before we have the answers we need.

Attempts to use other aspects of the pro- or anti-coagulation pathway to improve the predictive power of the conventional clotting tests have not so far gone beyond the stage of examining relatively small groups after the events, thus introducing additional variables (fibrinogen levels (10) and antithrombin (11, 12)).

(b) Fibrinolysis. On the basis of a theoretical and entirely unsubstantiated belief that in normal health the blood is maintained in a liquid flowing state because an active fibrinolytic system neutralises the clotting system (the concept of "natural fibrinolysis" - Astrup (13)) many workers have tried to compare the lytic activity or lytic capacity of various groups. Precisely the same problems of method and of group selection apply as in the clotting factor studies. Good examples of the earlier and current approach to the epidemiology of fibrinolysis are the "point-in-time" study in South Africa (7) and the more sophisticated, time-dependent longitudinal study of Meade (8, 14). Until the results of the latter study are available, we must regard the predictive potential of "natural fibrinolysis" as unproven.

Some workers have felt that the circulating blood might not be reflecting the lytic activity of the vessels themselves and over the years many studies have been performed on post-mortem and biopsy material using the fibrin-plate method (15). While vein biopsy is feasible, albeit invasive (16, 17) arterial biopsies are unlikely to find a place in the pre-symptomatic detection of potential vascular disease victims.

(c) Platelet behaviour. Because adherent platelets form a large part of the bulk of an arterial thrombus it is tempting to assume that the key to thrombus formation lies in an aberration of platelet behaviour. Two cautionary notes should be sounded; first, the platelets may be responding in a perfectly normal and appropriate way to some external message which one could not detect by examining the platelets themselves. An analagous situation would be the view obtained by passengers in a helicopter hovering over large towns on a Saturday afternoon and seeing huge masses of aggregated human beings clustering around a green rectangular area. Scooping up a section of these aggregates would reveal no consistent characteristic, and the clue would only come from examining the smaller number of brightly-coloured particles on the green area and from watching an even smaller particle move rapidly between them.

Second, unless one studies the living circulation, it is impossible to examine platelets without introducing a whole series of artefacts (venepuncture; contact with foreign surfaces; anticoagulation; centrifugation). In the circulation, the platelet is not exposed to any of these stimuli, and we should not assume that the tricks which platelets perform in vitro necessarily bear any direct relation to their activities in vivo. If we use the words "platelet behaviour in vitro" instead of "platelet function" we can regain our perspective. We must also remember that platelet behaviour is dependent on the concentration of the divalent cations calcium and magnesium, and that citrate, which is the most commonly used anticoagulant, may play a crucial part in determining the pattern of in vitro response (18, 19).

A bewildering array of "platelet function" tests have been used (20) and have given an equally diverse variety of results. The methods used include standardised bleeding time measurements (21), adhesion of platelets to glass or their entrapment in columns of glass beads (22, 23, 24), accretion of platelets on a filter (25, 26), platelet aggregation (22, 27, 28), survival time of isotopically-labelled platelets (29, 30, 31) and finally micro-electrophoresis (32). The latter test is time-consuming and is quite unsuited to any form of population screening, but it is interesting to note that Hampton and Gorlin (33) found that it gave an abnormal response pattern in 32 out of 34 patients with overt coronary disease and it was similarly abnormal in 17 out of 29 individuals who were completely well, but who were the first degree relatives of young men with coronary disease. It would be of interest to follow these 17, and the normal 12, over the years to see whether the test had predictive value.

As with the clotting and fibrinolytic systems, none of the platelet studies have been put to the predictive test. In many of them the inevitable difficulty of separating causes from consequences has arisen, and the overlap between "diseased" and "normal" subjects is considerable. The long term prospective study of initially healthy people previously mentioned (8) has included various tests of platelet behaviour in its data-base and the outcome of this study is awaited with interest. At the present time however, there is no test of platelet behaviour which can be used to separate individuals who will develop coronary disease from those who will not do so.

(d) Platelet-coagulation interactions. The role of material released from platelets in the initiation of blood clotting is well known (Platelet Factor 3) but three other platelet properties have recently engaged attention.

(1) "Platelet coagulant activities". The ability of platelets to influence coagulation in ways other than their traditional Factor 3 contribution have been described

by Walsh (34, 35, 36) under the generic heading of "platelet coagulant activities". Although no studies on the predictive value of this system have yet been reported in respect of coronary artery disease it is interesting to note that Walsh et al. (37) have studied 78 subjects, 22 of whom had transient cerebral ischaemic attacks, 18 of whom had other diseases and 38 of whom were normal. Twelve of the cerebro-vascular patients were found to have a two- to three-fold increase in their "platelet coagulant activities", while the other 10 were normal. This did not correlate with serum lipid levels, so it appeared that the test was picking out some other attribute. One should however, note that only half the group showed this attribute, so once more the discriminating power of the test for individuals is not high, nor has its predictive power been tested. Nevertheless, the inclusion of tests for "platelet coagulant activity" in long-term prospective studies would be of considerable interest.

(2) "Heparin neutralising activity". O'Brien (38, 39, 40, 41) has studied the ability of platelet-poor plasma to antagonise the action of added heparin. It seems likely that this heparin neutralising activity (HNA) derives from activated platelets and that it may be related to platelet factor 4. While there is no doubt that there is a profound change in HNA in patients who have sustained a myocardial infarction, the HNA then moves back towards normal as the acute illness resolves. Thus the mean clotting times which are used to measure HNA (a longer time indicating low HNA and a short time indicating high HNA) were 28.2 seconds in control subjects, and 12.8 seconds in patients with myocardial infarcts studied at 1-7 days. Over the succeeding period, the times returned towards normal (14.2 secs. at 8-28 days; 19.8 secs. at 1-3 months; 20.9 secs. in another group of patients studied at longer but unspecified intervals). The overlap between these post-infarction patients and the controls is indicated by the standard deviations of the means previously quoted (Controls 28.2 $\overset{+}{-}$ 6.01 seconds; post-infarction patients 20.9 $\overset{+}{-}$ 4.78 seconds). Thus the discriminatory power of the test for individual subjects is not high and its predictive value has not yet been determined.

(3) β-thromboglobulin. Moore et al. (42) described the isolation of a protein which seemed to originate from, and to be specific to platelets. Their hope was that if this material is released into the circulation when platelets participate in thrombus formation then altered levels of β-thromboglobulin would be detectable and would act as a marker for thrombosis. It has however, proved difficult to control all the variables and this must limit its value as a screening test (43). The venepuncture, the size of needle used and the vigour with which blood is expelled, the anticoagulant used, the time intervals and the temperatures used during storage and centrifugation, all contribute changes of sufficient magnitude to make it unlikely that smaller systematic differences between thrombosing and non-thrombosing subjects will be detectable.

Conclusions

In respect of conventional risk-factors, such as hyperlipidaemia, hypertension and cigarette smoking, Oliver (44) has commented "So far it has not been possible to predict who, in the apparently healthy population, will develop a heart attack ....
It is not possible also to differentiate, even within individuals with the highest category of risk, those who will develop a heart attack in the foreseeable future compared with those who will have no event during the next 10 years". Oliver went on to point out that even the highest risk category has poor predictive value. Thus, of a group of individuals who smoked, who had raised arterial pressure and raised plasma lipids, 92% survived 10 years without incident (Report of Inter-Society Commission (1970) (45). Conventional screening therefore only "predicted" correctly 8% of individuals within a 10 year follow-up period.

There must therefore be additional risk factors or risk markers which determined why 8 out of 100 did, and 92 out of 100 did not, develop heart attacks. Despite a size-

able investment of effort in the detection of potential markers of thrombosis, we
have no blood test which will add discriminating power to the existing risk factors.
This may be because thrombosis is not the prime mover in the clinical events which
we wish to forestall, because thrombosis is not due to, or accompanied by, detectable changes in the circulating blood or finally because there is a thrombotic marker but our in vitro tests cannot pick it up. Only time will resolve this dilemma,
but at the present time there is no blood test which can differentiate individuals
who will develop heart attacks from those who will not.

REFERENCES

(1) Rokitansky, C. (1852): A manual of pathological anatomy. Sydenham Society,
     London.
(2) Virchow, R. (1858): Die cellular Pathologie. Hirschwald, Berlin.
(3) Spain, D.M. and Bradess, V.A. (1960): Circulation, 22, 816.
(4) Baroldi, G., Radice, F., Schmid, G. and Leone, A. (1974): Am. Heart J., 87,
     65.
(5) McDonald, L. (1957): Br. Heart J., 19, 584.
(6) McDonald, L. and Edghill, M. (1958): Lancet, 1, 996.
(7) Merskey, C., Gordon, H. and Lackner, H. (1960): Br. Med. J., 1, 219.
(8) Meade, T.W. (1973): Thromb. Diath. Haem. Suppl. 54, 317.
(9) Meade, T.W., Brozovic, M., Chakrabarti, R., Howath, D.J., North, W.R.S. and
     Stirling, Y. (1976): Br. J. Haematol., 34, 353.
(10) Fulton, R.M. and Duckett, K. (1976): Lancet, 2, 1161.
(11) Innerfield, I., Stone, M.L., Mersheimer, W., Clauss, R.D. and Greenberg, J.
     (1976): Am. J. Clin. Pathol., 65, 384.
(12) Editorial: Long-term blood abnormalities in thrombosis (1973): Lancet, 2,
     133.
(13) Astrup, T. (1956): Blood, 11, 781.
(14) Meade, T.W., Chakrabarti, R. and North, W.R.S. (1976): Br. Med. J., 1, 837.
(15) Todd, A.S. (1959): J. Pathol. Bact., 78, 281.
(16) Rawles, J.M., Warlow, C. and Ogston, D. (1975): Br. Med. J., 2, 61.
(17) Browse, N.L., Gray, L., Jarrett, P.E.M. and Morland, M. (1977): Br. Med. J.,
     1, 478.
(18) MacFarlane, D.E., Walsh, P.N., Mills, D.C.B., Holmsen, H. and Day, H.G. (1975):
     Br. J. Haematol., 30, 457.
(19) Heptinstall, S. (1976): Thromb. Haemostas., 36, 208.
(20) Hampton, J.R. and Mitchell, J.R.A. (1976): Thrombosis. In Human Blood Coag-
     ulation, Haemostasis and Thrombosis, 2nd Ed. Edited by Rosemary Biggs. Oxf-
     ord, Blackwell Scientific Publications, pp. 536-556.
(21) O'Brien, J.R., Etherington, M., Jamieson, S., Klaber, M.R. and Ainsworth, J.F.
     (1973): Lancet, 1, 694.
(22) O'Brien, J.R. and Heywood, J.B. (1966): Thromb. Diath. Haemorrh., 16, 752.
(23) Bygdeman, S. and Wells, R. (1969): J. Atherosclerosis Res., 10, 33.
(24) Sjögren, A., Bottiger, L.E., Biorck, G., Wahlberg, F. and Carlson, L.A. (1970):
     Acta Med. Scand., 187, 89.
(25) Swank, R.L. (1968): Ser. Haemat., 12, 146.
(26) Hornstra, G., Lewis, B., Chait, A., Tuppeinen, O., Karvonen, M.J. and Vergroe-
     sen, A.J. (1973): Lancet, 1, 1155.
(27) Carvalho, A.C., Colman, R.W. and Lees, R.S. (1974): N. Engl. J. Med., 290,
     434.
(28) Johnson, M., Ramey, E. and Ramwell, P.W. (1975): Nature, 253, 355.
(29) Murphy, E.A. and Mustard, J.F. (1962): Circulation, 25, 114.
(30) Abrahamsen, A.F. (1968): Scand. J. Haematol., 5 (Suppl. 3), 1.
(31) Steele, P.P., Weily, H.S., Davies, H. and Genton, E. (1973): Circulation, 48,
     1194.
(32) Hampton, J.R. and Mitchell, J.R.A. (1974): Thromb. Diath. Haemorrh., 31, 204.
(33) Hampton, J.R. and Gorlin, R. (1972): Br. Heart J., 34, 465.

(34) Walsh, P.N. (1972): Br. J. Haematol., 22, 237.
(35) Walsh, P.N. (1972): Br. J. Haematol., 22, 393.
(36) Walsh, P.N. (1974): Blood, 43, 597.
(37) Walsh, P.N., Pareti, F.I. and Corbett, J.J. (1976): N. Engl. J. Med., 295, 854.
(38) O'Brien, J.R. (1974): Thromb. Diath. Haemorrh., 32, 116.
(39) O'Brien, J.R., Etherington, M., Jamieson, S., Klaber, M.R. and Lincoln, S.V. (1974): Thromb. Diath. Haemorrh., 31, 279.
(40) O'Brien, J.R., Etherington, M., Jamieson, S. and Lawford, P. (1974): Lancet, 2, 656.
(41) O'Brien, J.R., Etherington, M., Jamieson, S., Lawford, P., Sussex, J. and Lincoln, S.V. (1975): J. Clin. Pathol., 28, 975.
(42) Moore, S., Pepper, D.S. and Cash, J.D. (1975): Biochim. Biophys. Acta, 379, 360.
(43) Ludlam, C.A. and Cash, J.D. (1976): Br. J. Haematol., 33, 239.
(44) Oliver, M.F. (1976): Scott. Med. J., 21, 164.
(45) Report of the Inter-Society Commission for Heart Disease Resources. Primary prevention of the atherosclerotic diseases. (1970): Circulation, 42, A55.

QUANTITATIVE ANGIOGRAPHY[*]

David Blankenhorn

University of Southern California, Los Angeles, U.S.A.

Very early recognition of coronary heart disease can involve either assessment of coronary atherosclerotic lesions or assessment of some early consequence of these lesions upon myocardial function. This paper is concerned with quantitative athero-sclerosis assessment with particular emphasis on early, non-obstructive, relatively uncomplicated lesions. If atherosclerotic lesions can be recognized and stabilized at this stage, mortality from atherosclerosis should decline or be delayed.

Development of quantitative angiography should be considered to have two distinct arenas of endeavour; coronary vessels and all other vessels. With the exception of coronary arteries, vessels have pulsation and some additional minor movement, but really are fixed in position as subjects for assessment. The superficial femoral artery will be discussed as an example of a stationary vessel. Coronary arteries present a very difficult and quite different problem because of the gross dynamic movement of the heart. Coronary lesion assessment lags significantly behind what is possible in other vessels.

Femoral Atherosclerosis Assessment

Quantitative angiography for femoral atherosclerosis assessment involves modification of usual clinical techniques. These have been developed to provide information of immediate use in patient care and answers such questions as: Is blood flow obstruct-ed? What is the capacity of collateral circulation? Atherosclerosis assessment re-quires resolution of fine details in the vascular shadow and therefore must deal with relatively small image areas. There is a trade off between image size and resolut-ion. It follows that when a large area is included in the image, less fine detail is provided. A first step in quantitative angiography is to establish a realistic limit for the area included in the examination in view of the desired resolution. It is useful to locate vessel edges with a precision of 100 microns to evaluate femoral atherosclerosis. Therefore, it is only practical to evaluate approximately 20 linear centimeters in five centimeter units, although the ilio-femoral-popliteal system of potential interest can extend for more than one meter. Modification of conventional angiography for quantitative atherosclerosis assessment also requires uniform posit-ioning of patients, standardization of background film density, and use of a small focal spot X-ray source. A feasible routine procedure to obtain films of the requir-ed quality with conventional radiographic equipment has been published by Barndt and co-workers from this institution (1).

Computer assessment of femoral angiograms provides information correlated with what human readers obtain (1), but significantly more comprehensive (2). The system we employ, shown in Figure 1, consists of a Dicomed D-57 image dissector controlled by a PDP 11/45 computer. Figure 2 illustrates the mechanism of the image dissector. A vacuum tube contains a light sensitive face plate which "boils" electrons in proport-

[*] Supported by NHLBI Specialized Center of Research in Atherosclerosis; NASA Office of Life Science Program, Medical Image Analysis Facility; and the Robert E. and May R. Wright Foundation.

TABLE 1

REPEAT SCANNING AND COMPUTER ANALYSIS OF ONE FILM				
11 Tests; 12-5-75 to 2-26-76				
Date	R 3,21	R 97,321	TL 90	CEA	CEC
12-5	45	45	169	113	16
12-10	47	49	162	112	17
1-2	47	48	163	112	17
1-9	46	46	158	115	16
1-16	47	46	169	111	16
1-23	47	51	174	115	17
2-4	45	50	157	117	17
2-8	48	46	168	111	16
2-13	46	46	157	114	16
2-20	46	44	171	112	15
2-26	48	50	177	118	17
Mean	46.5	47.4	165.9	113.6	16.4
Standard Deviation	1.0	2.3	6.9	2.9	0.7
Coefficient of Variation	2.2%	4.9%	4.2%	2.1%	4.1%

R 3,21 = Roughness 3,21; TL 90 = Taper lumen 90; CEA = Computer Estimated
Atherosclerosis; and CEC = Computer Estimated Cholesterol conent.
See text for explanation.

ion to the intensity of light striking it. Electromagnetic coils deflect electrons through a pin hole to provide a signal proportional to densities throughout the image. The D-57 image dissector generates a sampling raster of 2,048 lines by 2,048 points to cover a film area of 54 x 54 mm. The minimum sample spacing is 0.026 mm. Using 0.052 mm spacing a typical femoral shadow 2.5 cm in width and 5 cm in length is converted into a 512 by 1024 digital array depicting up to 256 shades of grey. As scanning proceeds, the digitized image is recreated and displayed in 16 shades of grey to the computer operator on a television monitor.

Computer assessment of the digitized image begins with location of vessel edges. The vessel is oriented vertically in the field and search for edge points is along horizontal scan lines perpendicular to the vessel (Figure 3). Radiographic images are created by differential absorption of transmitted energy emitted from an X-ray source several hundred microns wide and "true" edge points with 1:1 correspondence to actual vessel lumen do not exist. We obtain an estimate of vessel edge location as follows: the density gradient of all points along each scan line is calculated as the derivative of a moving, second degree, least squares, polynomial centered on the point and fitted through 11 points on each side of it. The density profile of a typical horizontal scan line and the derived gradient plot is shown in Figure 4. Edges located by this measure can be used for atherosclerosis assessment and are attractive for visual presentation because plotted vessel edges are close to where human observers tend to expect them intuitively, Figure 5.

When vessel edges have been located, vessel irregularity is quantitated by two general classes of measures. The first class of measure derives information from the edge profile alone. These are procedures of choice when an image dissector is employed, Figure 6 illustrates one such measure. Two filters (moving averages) are applied sequentially along vessel edge points. The length of each filter determines the degree of vessel edge smoothing. Roughness is the root mean square difference between smoothing from a short filter and a long filter (Figure 7). Selection of different filters can tune measures to various lesion sizes. For example, a three point filter followed by a 21 point filter (R 3,21) removes some edge irregularity, but is sensitive to small plaques. A 91 point filter followed by a 321 point filter (R 91,321) is sensitive to larger plaques. Another measure deriving information from vessel edges is Lumen 90 with taper (TL90). To obtain this, left and right vessel edges are averaged to obtain a sequence of vessel midpoints. Taper is determined from the slope of a statistical regression line of vessel widths as a function of distance along the vessel. Midpoints are smoothed with a 401 point filter, corrected for taper, and translated to left and right until 90 per cent of all edge points are included. The root mean square difference between original edges and translated edges is Lumen 90 with taper, Figure 8. This measure can also be used without correction for vessel taper and is called Lumen 90 (L90). Edge measures are most sensitive to the presence of plaques when these occur in profile at the vessel edge.

The second class of measure derives information from optical densities between vessel edges. These measures are not influenced by rotation of the vessel, but are sensitive to image contrast variation that results from enface plaques. They sometimes perform erratically when an image dissector of the Dicomed D-57 type is used to sample the radiographic image. An exact description of individual and combined vessel measures of the type described above to estimate atherosclerosis severity (CEA-computer estimated atherosclerosis) or vessel wall cholesterol content (CEC-computer estimated cholesterol) is given in an autopsy study of human femoral artery by Crawford and co-workers at this institution (2).

Replication of scanning and computer analysis on the same film is shown in Table 1. The precision of measures varies from two to five per cent. The effect of varying contrast medium concentration and exposure conditions on computer assessment of an arterial cast is shown in Table 2. Coefficient of variation is from three to five

TABLE 2

		R 97,321			L90*			CEA			CEC	
	75	80 KVP	85	75	80 KVP	85	75	80 KVP	85	75	80 KVP	85
EFFECTS OF EXPOSURE AND CONTRAST CONCENTRATION ON COMPUTER MEASURES												
I_2 mg/ml												
48	147	159	142	534	553	539	214	203	197	45	49	44
97	147	141	148	506	520	493	209	209	207	45	43	45
145	147	144	148	491	493	505	205	210	219	45	45	45
194	141	146	144	474	489	473	209	214	217	43	45	44
242	143	143	144	486	480	508	210	217	219	44	44	44
Coefficient of Variation	2.9%			4.6%			2.9%			3.0%		

*L90 = Lumen 90. See text for explanation.

Other abbreviations are as in Table 1.

TABLE 3

PRECISION COMPARISON IN SEQUENTIAL FILMS FROM ONE ANGIOGRAM	
Six Patients, Two Films Each	
Measure	Coefficient of Variation
R 3,21	4.5%
R 81,97	4.4%
R 97,321	6.1%
L90	5.7%
TL90	3.9%
CEA	2.2%
CEC	4.6%

per cent. An estimate of the precision of the method during clinical use in man derived by comparing two sequential films from the same examination is shown in Table 3. The coefficient of variation is from two to six per cent.

Discrimination of specific lesion types may be possible by computer analysis of angiograms. Among 128 segments of femoral artery examined postmortem we identified seven as completely normal, six with uncomplicated stenosis, and 14 with hemorrhagic ulceration. The remaining 101 segments exhibited a heterogeneous group of lesions not readily assigned to any single classification. These were designated as unassigned. Table 4 illustrates the ability of a six step discriminant function to identify these lesions from each other. First a conventional discriminant analysis was used to distinguish among lesion types. Then a more conservative method, jackknife classification, was applied. The jackknife procedure misclassified one segment with hemorrhagic ulceration as uncomplicated stenosis. All other segments were correctly classified.

When serial angiograms are evaluated, a small degree of vessel rotation can mimic lesion change. This problem is avoided by measures which derive information from film densities between vessel edges. Crawford and co-workers have developed a method to reconstruct vessel profiles from these densities in a single plane angiogram (3). Figure 9 illustrates reconstruction of a femoral vessel with two opposing plaques. Both plaques were smaller when re-examined, after 13 months and the apparent change in size cannot be due to vessel rotation. Application of this method requires film with a proper range of densities and use of a precise scanning densitometer.

Coronary Atherosclerosis Assessment
The quality of images which can be obtained from coronary artery is less than can be obtained from other vessels of comparable size. Many of the reasons for this are related to cardiac motion. Coronary images are blurred except when exposure times are short. Unless very high milliamperage is used (2000 mA, which increases effective focal spot size) short exposure times limit the amount of radiation which can be passed through the chest. This in turn limits the amount of information obtainable by radiography. Cardiac motion produces intermittent overlapping of ribs and other coronary vessels and so there is continual change in background density and scattered radiation. The plane of the lumen of certain coronary vessels changes suddenly in relation to the image plane at irregular intervals during the cardiac cycle. This problem is particularly severe in the left main coronary segment.

Quantitative assessment of coronary angiograms is now at an early stage of development. Various reading procedures are being tested on films produced to meet clinical requirements. It is assumed (but not proven) that films of high quality for judging surgical prospects are also optimal for atherosclerosis assessment. All published coronary assessment methods are limited in precision to what can be achieved after a human locates the vessel edges, the majority rely on an observer to perform the entire process. The accuracy of independent film readers has been evaluated by comparing stenosis estimates with postmortem findings (4, 5, 6) and found reasonably acceptable in a qualitative sense - recognition of 50 per cent stenosis (6) or 75 per cent stenosis (4). Nonetheless, among 23 consecutive patients who died following coronary artery grafting within 30 days of a previous coronary cineangiogram, Grondin and co-workers identified four cases where failure to assess the degree of coronary arterial narrowing lead to incomplete myocardial revascularization (5).

The consistency of four highly experienced individual film readers was evaluated in quantitative terms by Zir and co-workers (7) who conclude "interobserver variability is a significant limitation to coronary angiography and clearly requires further study". DeRouen reports a study of 11 readers evaluating ten angiograms, "the aver-

TABLE 4

	COMPUTER DISCRIMINATION OF LESION TYPES		
Computer Measure	Initial Standard Classification % Correct	Jackknife Classification % Correct	Significance*
L90	81	78	0.001
Min./Ave. Width	85	78	0.001
R 21,33	89	81	0.05
R 41,49	100	89	0.01
R 81,97	100	96	0.01
R 21,65	100	96	0.05

*Significant at Step 6

TABLE 5

STANDARD DEVIATION OF STENOSIS ESTIMATION BY AN EXPERT FOUR MAN PANEL			
Left Main	24.8%	Obtuse Marginal	13.3%
Left Anterior Descending$_1$	7.0%	Posterolateral	14.5%
Left Anterior Descending$_2$	5.2%	Right Coronary Artery$_1$	3.2%
		Right Coronary Artery$_2$	2.1%
Left Anterior Descending$_3$	18.1%	Right Coronary Artery$_3$	3.8%
Diagonal$_1$	29.7%	Posterior Descending	17.3%
Diagonal$_2$	1.3%	Inferior Wall Branches	6.5%
Circumflex$_1$	9.1%		
Circumflex$_2$	11.1%		

age standard deviation for estimation of any segmental stenosis by a single reader was 18 per cent" (8). We have studied the consistency of a panel of expert angiographers* who evaluated 14 films twice at an interval of seven months (9). The panel working as a group required an average of 30 minutes to evaluate each film. The overall standard deviation of stenosis estimation was 14 per cent. The range of standard deviation in various arterial segments was 1 to 30 per cent (Table 5). The standard deviation of stenosis of left main coronary artery segment was 25 per cent. This appears noteworthy because Zir and co-workers also report "that in 3/20th (15 per cent) angiograms there was disagreement by at least one observer about the significance of lesions noted in the main left coronary artery". Further investigation of consistency and accuracy of left main segment evaluation should be given high priority because lesions in this location are of particular importance.

A logical next step in coronary atherosclerosis assessment appears to be augmentation of human film readers' interpretations with instrumental stenosis estimates. This should preserve intuitive value judgements where human interpreters exceed anything now possible with instruments, but provide assistance where humans perform poorly. Cranston and co-workers (10) examining sources of error in postmortem atherosclerosis assessment identified visual assessment of lesion area as a significant limitation. They found "planimetric measurement was reproducible, but visual assessment was extremely variable; it was shown that visual assessment of area is inaccurate as well as poorly reproducible. It was not possible to improve visual performance, or to correct its errors". Robbins and Rodriquez (11) studying postmortem coronary atherosclerosis by angiography came to similar conclusions.

A technique improving stenotic area estimation in coronary angiograms has been reported by Brown and co-workers (12). They have developed a computer program which estimates coronary stenosis from perpendicular angiographic projections after a human observer has traced the edges of each vessel to be measured with a light pen. With this procedure the standard deviation of per cent stenosis is reported to be less than 5 per cent in clinical films. An earlier, less sophisticated, technique developed by Gensini used adjustable cross-hairs to locate the position of vessel edges and measured average vessel width (13). What now should be done is to remove the element of human error further with instrumental means to locate vessel edges. Human observers have very limited ability to quantitate closely matched shades of grey. It is inherent in the process of angiography that edges of a vessel image are delineated by many shades of grey. An adaptation of femoral edge finding procedures to coronary vessel edges is shown in Figure 10 (14). The new procedure can follow curved vessels and is not limited to parallel scanning at right angles to the major axis of the vessel. With slight modification this new procedure is now being applied to retinal vessel photographs.

Image Averaging to Reduce Angiographic Risk and Discomfort
Assessment of atherosclerosis in any vascular bed will be most useful if it can be applied to patients with early lesions. The risks and discomforts of angiography now tend to limit this procedure to symptomatic individuals who usually have extensive atherosclerosis with lesions in late stages of development. Femoral angiography has the precision required to evaluate early atherosclerotic lesions and we

*
J. Michael Criley, M.D., Professor of Medicine and Radiology, UCLA School of Medicine; Melvin P. Judkins, M.D., Professor and Chairman, Department of Radiology, Loma Linda University School of Medicine; George G. Rowe, M.D., Professor of Medicine, University of Wisconsin School of Medicine; and Ronald H. Selvester, M.D., Professor of Medicine, University of Southern California School of Medicine.

would like to reduce the risk and discomfort to limits acceptable to asymptomatic subjects. It seems possible that contrast medium concentrations required for computer evaluated angiograms can be reduced through image averaging. We have reason to believe that amounts recommended for high dose excretion urography, 600 mg iodine/kg body weight by rapid intravenous injection (15) may be adequate. We have calculated the iodine concentrations present in femoral artery on first pass following intravenous injection using equations of Middleman (16) and Simon (17). If 100 ml of Hypaque 75 M^r is given in four seconds into the antecubital vein of a 70 kg man with normal resting cardiac output and central blood volume, peak iodine concentration in femoral artery will be 23 mg/ml. Eighty per cent of this peak concentration (18.5 mg iodine/ml) will be present in the femoral artery for five seconds, a period adequate to expose 30 films with conventional radiographic equipment. The standard deviation of edge location in superficial femoral artery containing 20 mg iodine/ml in a thigh of usual size is 400 microns (18). If 30 films are averaged, the standard deviation of edge finding should be 400/ 30 = 73 microns. If 20 films are averaged the standard deviation of edge finding should be 400/ 20 = 89 microns.

Results of a film averaging trial are shown in Table 6. A radiographic phantom immersed in six inches of water was filled with 14.5 mg iodine/ml. Ten serial films were exposed for 0.1 seconds each on a Schnonander changer with par speed screens. A rotating grid was employed and films were developed in an Xomat developer. Films were digitized after being aligned by hand on the image dissector. The error of edge finding in a single film was estimated by applying the R 3,21 measure and found to be 166. Table 6 compares the roughness found during sequential film averaging with that predicted by theory. When up to four films were averaged the reduction which occurred closely approximated that predicted by theory. When more films were averaged, the reduction found was less than predicted. We believe that small errors introduced by differences of film position due to hand mounting for digitization are the cause and may be corrected by mechanical registration procedures. The improvement in image quality by averaging in this first trial is illustrated in Figure 11 which compares a single film with averages of two, six and ten images. Image averaging appears to have greatest potential for atherosclerosis assessment in carotid and femoral vessels. It may provide means for precise lesion assessment with little risk and minimum discomfort to the subject.

TABLE 6

	REDUCTION OF EDGE FINDING ERROR BY IMAGE AVERAGING	
No. of Films Averaged (N)	Observed Measure R 3,21	Predicted Measure $\frac{166}{\sqrt{N}}$
1	166	166
2	115	117
4	84	83
6	77	68
8	76	59
10	69	52

REFERENCES

(1) Barndt, R., Jr., Blankenhorn, D.H., Crawford, D.W. and Brooks, S.H. (1977) :
Ann. Intern. Med., 86, 139.
(2) Crawford, D.W., Brooks, S.H., Selzer, R.H., Barndt, R., Jr., Beckenbach, E.S.
and Blankenhorn, D.H. (1977) : J. Lab. and Clin. Med., 89, 378.
(3) Crawford, D.W., Brooks, S.H., Barndt, R., Jr. and Blankenhorn, D.H. : Invest.
Radiol. (In Press).
(4) Schwartz, J.N., Kong, Y., Hackel, D.B. and Bartel, A.G. (1975) : Am. J. Cardiol., 36, 174.
(5) Grondin, C.M., Dyrda, I., Pasternac, A., Campeau, L., Bourassa, M.G. and
Lesperance, J. (1974) : Circulation, 49, 703.
(6) Vlodaver, Z., Frech, R., Van Tassel, R.A. and Edwards, J.E. (1973) : Circulation, 47, 162.
(7) Zir, L.M., Miller, S.W., Dinsmore, R.E., Gilbert, J.P. and Harthorne, J.W.
(1976) : Circulation, 53, 627.
(8) DeRouen, T.A., Murray, J.A. and Owen, W. (1977) : Circulation, 55, 324.
(9) Sanmarco, M.E., Brooks, S.H. and Blankenhorn, D.H. : Circulation (Submitted
for Publication).
(10) Cranston, W.I., Mitchell, J.R.A., Russell, R.W.R. and Schwartz, C.J. (1964) :
J. Athero. Res., 4, 29.
(11) Robbins, S.L. and Rodriquez, F.L. (1966) : Am. J. Cardiol., 18, 153.
(12) Brown, B.G., Bolson, E., Frimer, M. and Dodge, H.T. (1977) : Circulation, 55,
329.
(13) Gensini, G.G., Kelly, A.E., DaCosta, B.C.B. and Huntington, P.P. (1971) :
Chest, 60, 522.
(14) Selzer, R.H., Blankenhorn, D.H., Crawford, D.W., Brooks, S.H. and Barndt, R.,
Jr. (1976) : In: Proceedings of the Caltech/JPL Conference on Image Processing Technology, Data Sources and Software for Commercial and Scientific
Applications, California Institute of Technology, Pasadena, California,
November, 1976.
(15) Davies, P., Roberts, M.B. and Roylance, J. (1975) : Brit. Med. J., 2, 434.
(16) Middleman, S. (1972) : Transport Phenomena in the Cardiovascular System.
Wiley-Interscience, New York.
(17) Simon, W. (1972) : Mathematical Techniques for Physiology and Medicine.
Academic Press, New York.
(18) Crawford, D.W., Beckenbach, E.S., Blankenhorn, D.H., Selzer, R.H. and Brooks,
S.H. (1974) : Atherosclerosis, 19, 231.

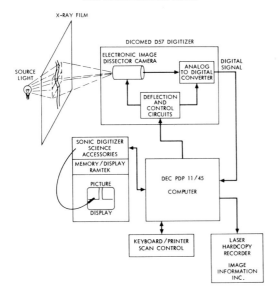

FIG. 1   Equipment for Image Processing of Angiograms.

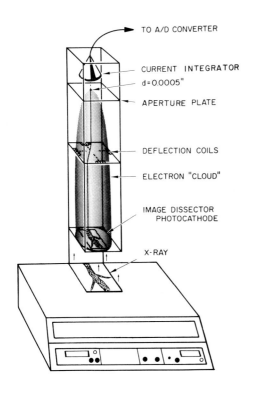

FIG. 2   The Mechanism of an Image Dissector.

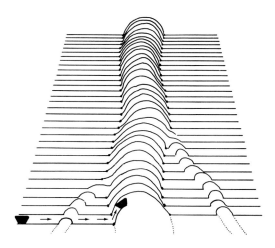

FIG. 3   Location of Vessel Edge Points by Search Along Horizontal Scan Lines.

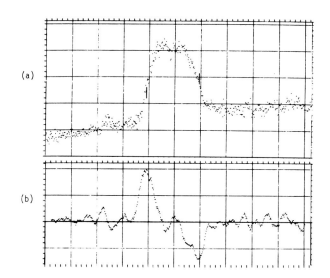

FIG. 4   Scan Line Analysis for Edge Detection.   (a) The density profile along one
scan line.   (b) Plot of the first derivative of (a).   Edges are located by
maximum and minimum points.

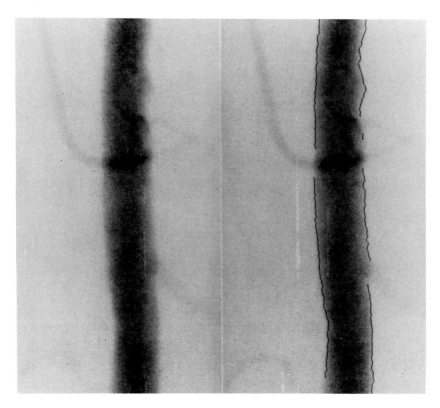

FIG. 5   A Femoral Vessel with Edge Points Located.   On the left a computer created
         image.   On the right the computer created image with edge points marked.

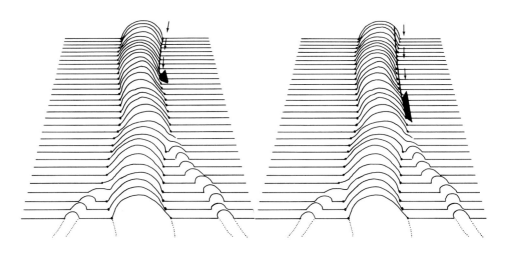

FIG. 6   Measuring Edge Roughness.   Two filters are applied sequentially down each
         vessel edge.

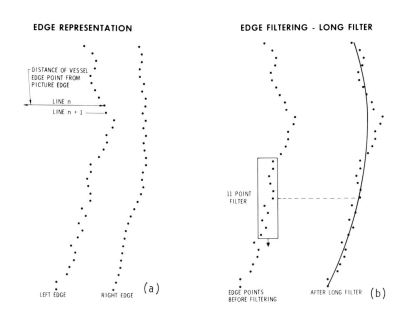

EDGE REPRESENTATION

DISTANCE OF VESSEL
EDGE POINT FROM
PICTURE EDGE

LINE n

LINE n + 1

LEFT EDGE   RIGHT EDGE   (a)

EDGE FILTERING - LONG FILTER

11 POINT
FILTER

EDGE POINTS
BEFORE FILTERING   AFTER LONG FILTER   (b)

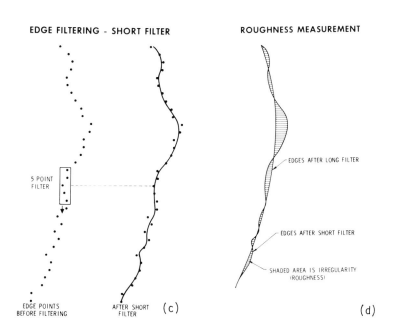

EDGE FILTERING - SHORT FILTER

5 POINT
FILTER

EDGE POINTS
BEFORE FILTERING   AFTER SHORT
FILTER   (c)

ROUGHNESS MEASUREMENT

EDGES AFTER LONG FILTER

EDGES AFTER SHORT FILTER

SHADED AREA IS IRREGULARITY
(ROUGHNESS)

(d)

FIG. 7   Comparison of Two Filters for Determining Edge Roughness. (a) Indicates
the vessel shadow before filtering; (b) Illustrates the effect of an 11
point filter on one vessel edge; (c) Illustrates the effect of a five point
filter on the same vessel edge; (d) Illustrates a graphic representation of
roughness measurement. The shaded area determines the magnitude of R 11,5.

39

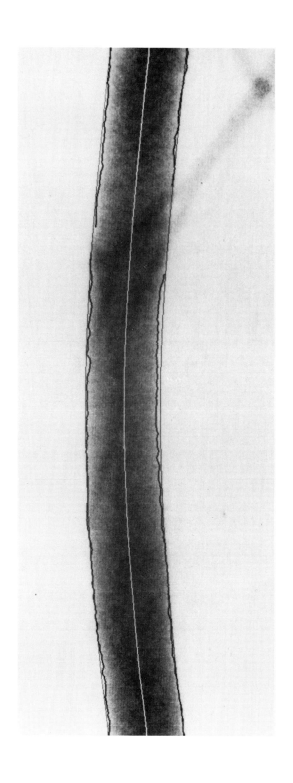

FIG. 8   A Femoral Vessel Image.   The Lumen 90 with taper measure has been applied.

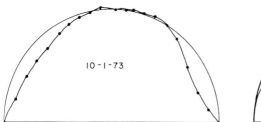 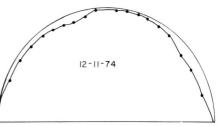

FIG. 9   Reconstruction of Vessel Profiles from Two Femoral Angiograms in the Same
Patient. On 10-1-73 plaque area on both sides of the vessel is indicated
by the difference between the found vessel profile (dotted line) and an
ideal round vessel (smooth line). On 12-11-74 plaque area has been reduced
on both sides of the vessel. Rotation of the vessel cannot be responsible
for this apparent reduction in size.

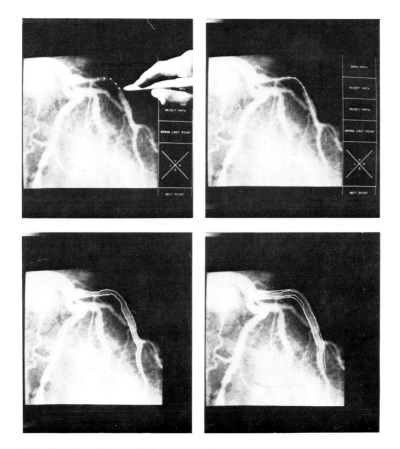

FIG. 10   Four Views of the Interactive Monitor During Coronary Edge Tracking. Upper
left: A light pen is used to place dots along the coronary artery to be
tracked. Upper right: The interactive monitor now displays a path for the
operator to inspect. If this path is accepted, edge finding will proceed
along scan lines perpendicular to it. Lower left: The operator has accepted the path and these vessel edges have been located. Lower right: Located vessel edges are next used for a L90 measurement which is displayed here.

41

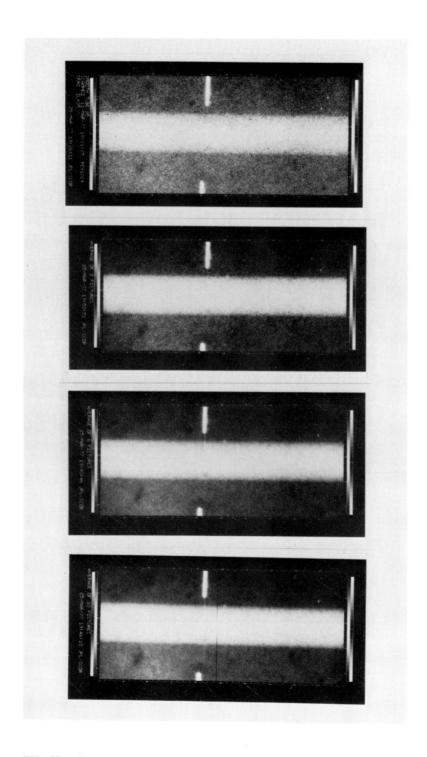

FIG. 11.   Improvement in Image Quality by Image Averaging. On the top a single
image; second from top the average of two images; third from top the
average of six images; and bottom the average of ten images.

NONINVASIVE IMAGING OF ATHEROSCLEROTIC LESIONS IN THE CAROTID ARTERIES OF PATIENTS

Bruce Kottke

Mayo Clinic, Rochester, Minnesota, U.S.A.

For many years it has been recognized that one of the major impediments to atherosclerosis research has been the lack of any noninvasive methods for measuring atherosclerotic plaques in living patients. Because of this handicap new therapeutic modalities can only be evaluated by massive clinical trials of many years' duration.
In these trials the frequency of complications is measured using "soft" endpoints.

While ideally one would prefer to measure coronary lesions noninvasively, a survey
of the state-of-the-art technology indicates that this may not be possible for quite
a few years. Since most of the biochemical and histologic features of coronary lesions are similar to those in the carotid and other peripheral arteries, it seemed
reasonable to assume that evaluation of lesions in these more accessible arteries
might provide a more useful indication of the effects of intervention manoeuvres than
can currently be obtained by large clinical trials.

To provide for the best possible resolution of images of lesions it seemed appropriate to concentrate on the carotid bifurcation initially and then extend the techniques to other peripheral arteries. This choice of strategy was based on the known
high incidence of lesions in this portion of the carotid artery and the fact that
with ultrasound B-scan techniques, resolution decreases rapidly as the distance from
the skin increases. In their attempt to formulate a programme for the development of
such an ideal instrument, investigators at Mayo sought an engineering group with a
high level of expertise in transducer design and techniques of ultrasound imaging.
It was our good fortune to obtain the collaboration of a very talented group of engineers headed by Mr. Phillip Green of Stanford Research Institute. In May of 1972, a
joint proposal to develop a high resolution, real time ultrasonic imaging technique
for the noninvasive assessment of atherosclerotic vascular disease was submitted to
National Institutes of Health.

Goals and Objectives of the Programme
The objectives of this Programme were:
(1) To develop a clinically practical real time ultrasound imaging system for the
     graphic display of arterial lesions and blood flow characteristics.
(2) To evaluate this instrument in normal and atherosclerotic carotid and femoral
     arteries in vivo in patients.
(3) To develop a quantitative system for on-line analysis and three dimensional
     display of ultrasonic data using advanced electronic signal processing and
     digital techniques.

Most of the first and second objectives have already been achieved. Planning is well
along for accomplishing the third objective over the next several years. Initially,
a prototype laboratory instrument was built at Stanford Research Institute and tested
at Mayo. From the experience gained with this prototype instrument, a second clinical version of the instrument was recently built and is currently undergoing clinical
evaluation in the study of patients at Mayo.

Description of the Clinical Instrument
The clinical instrument utilizes a 10 megahertz transducer with a lens which presents

an image of a 3 x 3 cm square region of tissue at a repetition rate of 15 frames/ second. The instrument was designed to display a blood velocity profile superimposed on this image generated by a 20-range gate pulsed Doppler subsystem operating at a frequency of 5 megahertz. The transducer is coupled to the patient via a small water bag and a mineral oil based coupling fluid. Pressure in the water bag is kept at 2 cm of water which is well below venous pressure to avoid any compression of the carotid artery. By turning the transducer assembly, images of both longitudinal and cross-sectional tissue planes of the vessels can be studied.

The instrument is designed so that images can be directly visualized, recorded on video tape or recorded on still Polaroid photographs. The still photos and playbacks of video tape recordings permit detailed evaluation at a later date and facilitate comparison of the results of ultrasound imaging with the results obtained by angiography.

Atherosclerotic lesions appear as a light shading within the black lumen of the vessel. By adjusting the transducer position, it is possible to select the longitudinal or cross-sectional plane that best portrays a particular lesion. In the majority of patients it is possible to easily visualize the carotid bulb, the bifurcation and the first portions of the internal and external carotid arteries. In about 5% of the patients such visualization is not possible because of problems with overlying obesity or a very short neck. The most common lesion sites are at the bifurcation near the origin of the internal and external branches. The longitudinal scans appear quite similar to angiograms except that they represent views of individual tissue planes rather than a compressed three dimensional image as is the case with angiography. The longitudinal sections cover a large area of the artery and are readily supplemented with cross-sectional views. The real time feature of the instrument greatly facilitates the recognition and identification of artifacts.

Early Experience with Patient Studies
Early clinical experience with the instrument demonstrated that the jugular vein is readily seen with the scanner and its pulsations can easily be appreciated. In addition, by having the patient do a Valsalva's manoeuvre or a Müller's manoeuvre it is very easy to see the rapid increase in diameter of the jugular vein with the Valsalva's manoeuvre and the collapse of the vein following the Müller's manoeuvre. These manoeuvres readily distinguish images of veins from images of arteries. Also because of the real time feature of the instrument it is easy to appreciate differences of arterial elasticity in young and old patients by observing the amplitude of the carotid artery pulsations. Obviously, the application of quantitative measures to these types of observations may be of use in the future in evaluating the function of arterial elastic tissue.

With the current instrument visualization of the femoral artery has been limited to the area just below the inguinal ligament. With further development of a variable focus system it is hoped that deeper portions of this vessel will eventually be seen.

The visualization of atherosclerotic lesions in the carotid artery with this instrument has exceeded our original hopes and expectations. Even relatively small lesions down to 1 mm in size have been visualized. By looking at the lesion in multiple planes in both longitudinal sections and at cross-sectional views and noting the movement of lesions with arterial pulsations, artifacts are readily separated from lesions and the full extent of the lesion can be readily appreciated. In heavily calcified lesions the more distal portion of the lesions may not be visualized because of a failure of ultrasonic waves to penetrate the dense calcification. This situation is readily recognized by the obvious shadow cast on the background signal by these dense lesions. In fact, these shadows have proven to be an important and helpful clue to the presence of lesions. In less calcified soft lesions, however, no shadow may be seen.

In some normal arteries a double wall reflection of normal carotid arteries is frequently noted. This finding is present primarily in older individuals and occasionally in young individuals with insulin-requiring diabetes mellitus. We have noted a very high correlation between the angiographic and ultrasonic differentiation of normal and abnormal arteries. In fact, this correlation exceeds 90%. In order to further evaluate the accuracy of the instrument in the detection of lesions, a small comparison study has been completed. In this study blinded observers interpreted the angiograms of 12 carotid arteries in 10 patients as well as the video tapes of ultrasonic evaluations of these same lesions. The interpretation was made on the basis of recording the number of stenoses or lesions seen and the degree of stenosis produced by each lesion. The compared angiograms and ultrasound B-scans were given dissimilar identification numbers and evaluated randomly by four physicians including a vascular radiologist, a vascular neurologist and two cardiovascular internists. Employing double-blind evaluation methods for the interpretations, the correlations of the interpretation of ultrasound B-scans with that of angiograms of the same arteries revealed a correlation coefficient of 0.897, a slope of 0.953 and a P value of 0.001. It is our suspicion that this less than 90% correlation between these two methods reflects the difficulties of interpretation of both the angiographic pictures and the ultrasound pictures. In certain isolated instances it appeared that the ultrasound approach had clear advantages over angiography. Smaller lesions and multiple lesions were often more readily imaged and made apparent by the B-scan images. The ultrasonic B-scans also had a distinct advantage when lesions were not seen in profile, but obscured by the superposition of dye on the angiogram. The limitations of the B-scans included unsuitability in the immediate postoperative period when raised skin scars were present and the fact that technically poor results were obtained in obese patients. With the present instrument the resolution of deeper arteries does not approach that usually obtained with angiography. Early experience indicates that dacron grafts can readily be distinguished from the native artery with the ultrasonic technique. In addition, in a few instances false hematomas at graft suture lines have been detected. In one instance a hematoma secondary to a carotid artery puncture has been identified. This appeared as a very soft lesion and was quite distinct in appearance from the typical atherosclerotic lesions seen in the artery. In several instances buckled carotid arteries were readily visualized and distinguished from carotid artery aneurysms using the ultrasonic technique.

A bonus finding in these studies has been the distinctive appearance of a normal thyroid gland as seen by ultrasound scanning. Small cysts and nodules as small as 5 mm in diameter have been clearly identified in the thyroid. Recently parathyroid tumours in a few patients have also been visualized. These tumours were subsequently proven at surgery. The limitations of these ancillary applications of the instrument have not, as yet, been fully defined. However, we are pursuing these potential applications as well as the arterial applications.

Summary
Over the next several years major emphasis of this development programme will be placed on the further evaluation of the Doppler subsystem and the development of digital processing techniques for reconstruction of three dimensional images by combining multiple longitudinal and cross-sectional scans. Hopefully, this will provide us a tool for the precise determination of lesion size. The availability of such a technique will be extremely useful for determining the effect of intervention treatments on lesion progression. Our ultimate goal is to use the instrument to document lesion regression.

INITIAL EVENTS IN ATHEROGENESIS

Colin Schwartz

Cleveland Clinic, Cleveland, Ohio, U.S.A.

Attempts to reconstruct a dynamic picture of the atherogenic sequence from either the complex morphology or chemical composition of the end-stage fibrous plaque have thus far been relatively disappointing. As a result, it has become increasingly apparent that we must both identify and describe the earliest stages of lesion development as a prelude to any decisive understanding of aetiological or pathogenic mechanisms. One potentially rewarding approach to this problem has been the information obtained from an exploration of the Evans Blue model. This model has consistently permitted the in vivo delineation of areas of spontaneously-differing endothelial permeability, arterial lipid metabolism and accumulation, and endothelial and intimal fine structure, differences which are demonstrable prior to lesion development.

The Evans Blue Model

Evans Blue, a protein-binding azo dye (T-1824) is known to complex tightly with normal serum albumin in the ratio of 1 molecule of dye to some 11 - 13 molecules of albumin (1). However, dissociation of this complex may occur in tissues (2) and in all likelihood accounts for the striking concentration of dye observed in the aortic intima in contrast to the distribution of ^{131}I-albumin across the full thickness of the aortic media. Notwithstanding the various implications of dissociation of the albumin-dye complex, the aortic uptake of Evans Blue exhibits a consistent and focal pattern in the dog (3), rabbit (4) and the pig (5 - 7) in vivo, a pattern not reproducible in vitro (8). Both the focal nature of the dye uptake, and the failure to reproduce the in vivo pattern in vitro have together been interpreted as reflecting the importance of focal differences or disturbances in aortic hemodynamics (8, 9). The latter possibility has been further validated by the observation that experimental aortic coarctation significantly modifies the spontaneous patterns of in vivo aortic dye uptake (9). In Figure 1 the normal or spontaneous pattern of aortic dye uptake in the young pig (Figure 1a) is compared with that resulting from post-ductal aortic coarctation (Figure 1b). In the healthy young pig (Figure 1a) dye uptake is most extensive in the thoracic aorta, and is characteristically located near the brachiocephalic branches, within the sinuses of Valsalva, and in close proximity to the obliterated ductus scar. Distally, smaller and less intense areas of bluing are seen at or near the intercostal, renal, or mesenteric ostia, and the flow dividers of the aortic trifurcation. Aortic coarctation (Figure 1b) results in an increased area and intensity of dye uptake in the arch proximal to the coarctation, together with decreased bluing distally.

The role of fluid dynamic factors in arterial transport and atherogenesis has been the subject of a number of studies or reviews (10 - 16). Fry (10 - 12) has shown in acute experiments that the arterial uptake of Evans Blue is increased with increased pressure or wall strain, increased shearing stress, and with turbulence. He has established that shearing stress of the order of 200 - 400 dynes/cm^2 at the blood vascular interface may result in endothelial injury or denudation, and further, that dye uptake may be increased before prominent endothelial injury has occurred.

Clarification of the relationship of sites of spontaneously-occurring in vivo dye uptake to sites of subsequent atheromatous lesion development is of considerable importance. McGill et al. (3) noted that areas of Evans Blue accumulation in the canine

TABLE 1

Time Post-Injection	Permeability Area	Vesicles / u^2 Endothelium	% Vesicles with FE	FE Grains / Vesicle
		UPTAKE OF FERRITIN BY AORTIC ENDOTHELIUM IN THE EVANS BLUE MODEL		
1 Min	White	39.7	10.3	1.0
	Blue	25.7	22.1*	1.1
5 Min	White	18.7	4.6	2.2
	Blue	17.9	12.5*	2.9
15 Min	White	24.9	12.0	0.9
	Blue	36.1	21.1*	1.3
Average	White	27.8	9.0	1.4
	Blue	26.6	18.6*	1.8

*$p < 0.05$

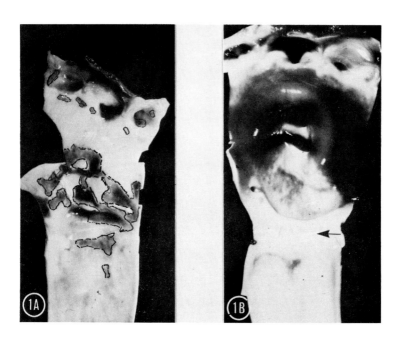

FIG. 1   Figure 1a to the left shows the thoracic aorta of a young pig 3 hours after the administration of Evans Blue. On the right (1b) we see the influence of post-ductal coarctation on the dye uptake pattern. The level of the line of coarctation is arrowed.

aorta delineate foci destined to develop atheromatous lesions. Fry (12) has confirmed these observations, indicating that in both the dog and pig, the pattern of dye
uptake is "virtually identical to the pattern of sudanophilia in early experimental
atherosclerosis". These conclusions are consistent with our own experience with the
distribution of spontaneously-occurring aortic lesions in the elderly pig, and the
greater accumulation of cholesterol and cholestryl esters in areas of dye uptake
(blue areas) relative to areas of no dye uptake (white areas) in the cholesterol-fed
pig (17, 18).

Endothelial Permeability
Enhanced endothelial permeability to macromolecules, including lipoproteins, is, we
believe, the essential initial event in the atherogenic sequence. Specifically,
sites destined to develop atheroma, as delineated by the in vivo uptake of Evans
Blue, have been established as areas of greater permeability, both to radio-iodinated
albumin, and also to the much larger fibrinogen molecule (19, 20). Figure 2 summar-
izes the results of a series of experiments in which ^{131}I-albumin uptake was studied.
For simplicity ^{131}I-albumin uptake has been expressed as a percentage, taking the
value for white areas in the thoracic aorta as 100%. Not only is the uptake significantly greater in thoracic blue relative to thoracic white areas, (Figure 2), but
regional differences can also be discerned, with uptake in the upper or lower abdom-
inal segments significantly less than in blue or white areas in the thoracic aorta.
With the much larger fibrinogen molecule, similar uptake patterns have emerged
(Figure 3). Both ^{131}I-albumin and ^{131}I-fibrinogen also exhibit distinct transmural
aortic gradients, with activity greatest in the intima and inner media, and least in
the outer media (Figures 4 and 5). These gradients indicate that most albumin or
fibrinogen has entered the aorta through the endothelium and that the blue-white uptake and gradient differences do indeed reflect differences in aortic endothelial
permeability to proteins. This influx of fibrinogen in the normal aorta is consistent with the observations of Smith et al. (21) and Smith (22) who, on the basis of
the recovery of soluble fibrinogen-fibrin antigen from normal human intima and early
fibrous lesions have concluded that substantial amounts of plasma fibrinogen enter
the intima.

The presence of fibrinogen or fibrin in arterial fatty streaks or atheromatous plaques has in the past been interpreted as evidence for a thrombogenic pathogenesis (23).
A number of studies have also demonstrated the occurrence of material antigenically
similar to fibrin or fibrinogen in both fatty streaks and atheromatous plaques (24,
27). But the diffuse distribution of fluorescence (25, 27) and the absence of demonstrable platelet antigenic material (27, 28) in early or uncomplicated lesions has
questioned the thrombotic origin of all plaque fibrin, a conclusion supported by our
data which indicate that at least some of the fibrin/fibrinogen in early lesions may
be explained on the basis of spontaneous endothelial permeability to fibrinogen (20).

It is of some interest that in the young pig, aortic endothelial permeability to ^{131}I-
albumin is increased almost 2-fold after only a short period on a cholesterol-supplemented diet, and prior to lesion development. A similar increase in endothelial
permeability has been observed in the cholesterol-fed rabbit (29). A spectrum of
subtle fine structural changes accompany this increased endothelial permeability (30),
including leucocyte adhesion, increased numbers of lysosomes and cytoplasmic filaments
within the endothelium, and an excess of blood-derived cells in the intima.

Apart from the permeability studies with isotopically-labelled proteins described
above, the magnitude and routes of trans-endothelial transport in sites of differing
susceptibility to atheroma have been studied at the ultrastructural level employing
ferritin (diameter 110Å), as a particulate probe. Preliminary studies indicate that
the enhanced permeability of blue areas to ferritin relates not to the number of
pinocytotic vesicles, nor to the ferritin-carrying capacity of each vesicle, but to
the number of vesicles actively involved in the transport process (Table 1). This

TABLE 2

INCORPORATION OF [^{14}C]-OLEIC ACID INTO LIPID FRACTIONS OF
THE CHOLESTEROL-FED PIG AORTIC INTIMA (6 WEEKS)

(CPM/μG DNA/10^6 CPM IN INCUBATION MEDIUM)

	TOTAL LIPID	PHOSPHOLIPID	TRIGLYCERIDE	CHOLESTERYL ESTER
THORACIC BLUE	7.95**	4.92**	1.44**	0.64*
THORACIC WHITE	3.42	2.10	0.64	0.19
ABDOMINAL WHITE	3.69	2.40	0.70	0.15

** $p < 0.01$
* $p < 0.05$

TABLE 3

INCORPORATION OF [^{14}C]-OLEIC ACID INTO INDIVIDUAL PHOSPHOLIPIDS
OF CHOLESTEROL-FED PIG AORTIC INTIMA (6 WEEKS)

(CPM/MG DNA/10^6 CPM IN INCUBATION MEDIUM)

	SPHINGOMYELIN	LECITHIN	PHOSPHATIDYL INOSITOL	PHOSPHATIDYL ETHANOLAMINE
THORACIC BLUE	0.063	3.27**	0.97*	0.61*
THORACIC WHITE	0.016	1.36	0.44	0.28
ABDOMINAL WHITE	0.018	1.55	0.49	0.33

** $p < 0.01$
* $p < 0.05$

concept of active or inactive vesicles suggests either that there is more than one type of vesicle, or alternatively, that activation of vesicles may be subject to regulatory control. Additionally, one should comment that aortic endothelial transport of ferritin is exclusively vesicular with no involvement of the intercellular junctions (Figure 6).

Vesicular transport is a process whereby plasma molecules enter "caveolae intracellulares" or invaginations on the luminal plasma membrane. These caveolae bud off into the cytoplasm to become pinocytotic vesicles ranging in size from 400 - 1500 Å diameter, which move from the luminal to the abluminal surface, a process which is summarized schematically in Figure 7. Movement may be bidirectional. In terms of atherogenesis, low density lipoprotein (diameter- 220Å) could, on the basis of molecular size, readily enter the caveolae and move across the endothelium in pinocytotic vesicles, a process less likely for the larger VLDL and chylomicrons. Factors regulating or controlling vesicular transport are poorly understood, and pose one of the more important research questions for the future. Specifically, we need more precise information on the roles of hypertension, vasoactive compounds, - including angiotensin and the prostaglandins, - and the pathophysiological significance of the endothelial glycocalyx or surface coat. The latter is readily visualized with the electron dense stain ruthenium red (31, 32). Areas of greater permeability and lesion susceptibility exhibit a glycocalyx which is some 2 - 5 fold thinner than areas of lesser permeability (32). It is tempting to suggest that the thicker glycocalyx over the latter areas might in part account for the lesser permeability, either by limiting access of molecules to plasmalemmal surface receptors or pinocytotic vesicles.

One potentially important alternative to vesicular transport must be considered, - namely injury to the endothelium with denudation of microscopic foci of cells resulting in the development of "ultra large pores", with loss of regulatory control of transendothelial transport. Some aspects of endothelial injury will be described subsequently.

Early Biochemical Events
Thus far we have briefly reviewed some aspects of the Evans Blue model which permits the identification of areas within the aorta destined to develop atheroma months or years later. These areas of enhanced permeability (5, 19, 20, 33) exhibit a number of other important features, including altered lipid metabolism, increased endothelial cell turnover, and numerous morphological differences (32, 33, 35). While it is likely that the underlying medial metabolic anomalies in these susceptible areas result from the greater influx of plasma constituents, the mechanisms have yet to be established.

Although pre-lesion (blue) areas in the young normocholesterolemic pig have a cholesterol content comparable to that of white areas (6, 7) after periods of 6 or 16 weeks on a cholesterol-supplemented diet they exhibit a significant accumulation of cholesterol (17) in the intima and inner media (Figure 8). Additionally the incorporation of ^{14}C-oleic acid into total lipid, phospholipid, triglycerides and cholesteryl ester is significantly greater in blue than in white areas (Table 2). The greater incorporation of oleate into intimal cholesterol esters of pre-lesion areas is of considerable significance, as cholesteryl oleate is the ester which preferentially accumulates in atheromatous lesions (36, 37). Oleate also exhibits a significantly greater incorporation into intimal lecithin, phosphatidyl inositol, and phosphatidyl ethanolamine of blue relative to white areas (19), as summarized in Table 3.

Many additional aspects of lipid metabolism and biosynthesis have been described for pre-lesion (blue) and non-lesion (white) areas. Unesterified ^{3}H-cholesterol uptake has been shown to be significantly greater in blue than in white areas (Figure 9), and moreover to exhibit distinct transmural aortic gradients as early as 10 minutes after injection of the labelled cholesterol (Figure 10). The uptake of ^{3}H-unesteri-

fied cholesterol in all likelihood is largely the result of a non-energy-dependent
physico-chemical exchange (38). This greater exchange of cholesterol in blue relative to white areas may possibly reflect a greater plasmalemmal membrane area available for exchange. Whether an exchange process of this type can under certain circumstances be converted to a net influx, is an important question which has yet to be
answered.

Although the phospholipid content of blue and white areas derived from the normal-fed
young pig aorta is not measurably different (39), some differences in phospholipid
synthesis have been observed between these areas with $1-^{14}$C-acetate, but not with
^{14}C-U-glucose as precursors (40). With acetate, a significant proportion of the lab-
el incorporated appeared in phosphatidyl choline and sphingomyelin (40). This greater phospholipid synthesis in blue areas has one likely explanation, namely greater
membrane synthesis, probably reflecting a higher rate of cell injury and repair in
blue relative to white areas (34).

While one could consider many other aspects of lipid metabolism, one additional difference between pre-lesion and non-lesion areas deserves comment. With both $1-^{14}$C-
acetate and ^{14}C-U-glucose as precursors, it has been demonstrated that the incorporation into certain lipid fractions is enhanced by insulin at physiological concentrations (25 μ U/ml) in non-lesion or white areas, but not in pre-lesion or blue areas
(41, 42). This difference in insulin-regulated lipogenesis between sites of differing susceptibility to atherogenesis may reflect either inherent differences in insulin receptors, or the possibility that lipogenesis in blue areas is already maximally
stimulated. The findings may also point towards a link between atherogenesis and
diabetes mellitus, but at this point the mechanisms and ultimate significance of
these observations are uncertain. In these and in all such in vitro studies, interpretation should be tempered with caution because of the potential influence of disturbed endothelial integrity on intima-media metabolism (43).

Morphological Correlates of Early Lesion Development
Pre-lesion (blue) areas in the young healthy pig exhibit a significantly greater
endothelial cell turnover relative to contiguous non-lesion (white) areas as determined by ^{3}H-thymidine autoradiography (34). Expressed in terms of relative percentages, endothelial cell turnover is 137% and 100% in pre-lesion and non-lesion areas
respectively. The greater turnover in pre-lesion areas is considered to reflect
continuing focal haemodynamic injury at these sites. That the pre-lesion (blue)
areas are indeed sites of increased spontaneously-occurring endothelial cellular injury and death has been directly established both in silver-stained Haütchen preparations (Figure 11) and by electron microscopy (Figure 12). Pre-lesion areas exhibit
many fine structural differences relative to the non-lesion or white areas, including
a prominent subendothelial oedema, cuboidal endothelial cells with short intercellular junctions and few interdigitations, and a 2 - 5 fold thinner surface coat or glycocalyx (32). With silver-stained en-face preparations, many additional morphological differences have been observed (35) including frequent discontinuities or gaps in
the consistently thicker cell boundaries of pre-lesion areas, together with foci of
less distinct cellular polarity. The presence of intensely silver-stained dead or
injured cells in pre-lesion areas has already been alluded to. These occur with a
frequency of 2.91% in pre-lesion as compared to 0.71% in non-lesion areas, and provide
the morphological basis for a theoretical "ultra large pore" system supplementing the
significantly greater vesicular transport of macromolecules to the sub-endothelium
and media in pre-lesion areas.

Pre-lesion areas exhibit several other characteristics of potential importance.
First, they are more prone to develop severe endothelial injury after endotoxin (E
coli) administration than non-lesion areas (44) and second, they are also more susceptible to develop a spectrum of endothelial ultrastructural changes, including injury, after even short periods (2 - 6 weeks) on a cholesterol-lard diet (30). Figures

13 and 14 illustrate one such feature, namely the adherence of blood monocytes to
aortic endothelium 2 weeks after initiation of the diet. Additionally, it is of interest that anti-platelet serum to a very large extent prevents the development of
endotoxin-induced endothelial injury, suggesting that under certain circumstances
platelets may mediate the development of endothelial injury.

Pathogenic Mechanisms
Up to this point we have reviewed some features of the Evans Blue model which we consider facilitates the identification and examination of sites destined to develop
atheroma. There remain, however, many facets of the aetiology and pathogenesis which
have not been discussed. This section is devoted to such a discussion, albeit briefly.

Foci of enhanced endothelial permeability to macromolecules are an essential and
initial event in the atherogenic sequence, being responsible for the distinct distribution of lesions (45, 46). Such focal increases in permeability may result either from frank endothelial injury or from increased vesicular transport. While focal
hemodynamic disturbances probably contribute directly to the development of endothelial injury, an indirect mechanism, dependent upon the platelet-release reaction at or
near the endothelial surface may also prove to be of importance, if not in initiating
injury, then in enhancing it. In this context, the secretory release of certain
platelet constituents including 5-hydroxytryptamine, angiotensin, prostacyclin,
thromboxane A_2 lysosomal enzymes, and a permeability-inducing cationic protein is of
particular relevance. Other factors may contribute to endothelial injury or enhanced
macromolecular transport including hypertension, hyper-beta-lipoproteinaemia, immune
complex deposition, cigarette smoking and/or carbon monoxide, and a spectrum of
pharmacological compounds.

Platelets, apart from their possible role in the development of endothelial injury,
contain a relatively low molecular weight protein which enhances the growth of stationary phase arterial smooth muscle cells in culture (47, 48). This platelet growth
factor is considered to be important in atherogenesis (47, 48) as smooth muscle-like
cells are numerically predominant in atheroma, and may give rise not only to lipid-
rich foam cells, but are also responsible for the secretion of collagen and elastin.
Many other "compounds" can stimulate mammalian cell growth in culture (49 - 51). To
conclude that platelet growth factor is the critical or sole mitogen in atherogenesis
is probably scientifically premature, particularly as low density lipoprotein has
also been shown to enhance smooth muscle cell proliferation (52, 53) and monotypic
cell growth in human plaques is considered to be monoclonal in nature on the basis of
glucose-6-phosphate-dehydrogenase isoenzyme studies (54 - 56).

Other basic molecular biological aspects of atherogenesis have emerged in recent
years, including the concept of atheroma as a lysosomal storage disease (57). Equally important has been the development of an understanding of the nature of membrane
receptor mechanisms to lipoproteins and the biology of lipoprotein endocytosis (58,
59).

Postscript
It is not possible nor even desirable to attempt to examine every facet of atherogenesis in this paper. Clearly, we have adopted the view that increased endothelial permeability is the initial event, due either to altered vesicular function or frank cellular injury, resulting in the enhanced focal influx of macromolecules such as low
density lipoproteins into the subendothelium and media. Subsequent complex interactions between initiating and accelerating factors, notably platelets, platelet constituents and low density lipoprotein result in plaque growth, and eventually in the
clinically significant complication, thrombotic occlusion.

Summary

Morphological and biochemical features occurring in pre-lesion areas delineated by the in vivo arterial uptake of the protein-binding azo-dye Evans Blue have been described. These areas, destined to develop atheroma, exhibit an increased permeability to proteins, enhanced endothelial cell turnover, lipid accumulation, and a variety of differences in lipid biosynthesis relative to non-lesion areas. Lipid biosynthesis in pre-lesion (blue) areas is not influenced by insulin, in contrast to the stimulatory effects observed in non-lesion or white areas. On the basis of ferritin studies, it is concluded that in pre-lesion areas enhanced vesicular transport is occurring. The significance of these findings in terms of atherogenesis are discussed and reviewed.

REFERENCES

(1) Rawson, R.A. (1943): Amer. J. Physiol., 138, 708.
(2) Stoelinga, G.B.A. and Van Munster, P.J.J. (1967): Acta Physiol. Pharmacol. Neerl., 14, 391.
(3) McGill, H.C., Geer, J.C. and Holman, R.L. (1957): Arch. Path., 64, 303.
(4) Friedman, M. and Byers, S.O. (1963): Arch. Path., 76, 99.
(5) Packman, M.A., Rowsell, H.C., Jørgensen, L. and Mustard, J.F. (1967): Exp. Molec. Pathol., 7, 214.
(6) Somer, J.B. and Schwartz, C.J. (1971): Atherosclerosis, 13, 293.
(7) Somer, J.B. and Schwartz, C.J. (1972): Atherosclerosis, 16, 377.
(8) Bell, F.P., Somer, J.B., Craig, I.H. and Schwartz, C.J. (1972): Atherosclerosis, 16, 369.
(9) Somer, J.B., Evans, G. and Schwartz, C.J. (1972): Atherosclerosis, 16, 127.
(10) Fry, D.L. (1968): Circ. Res., 22, 165.
(11) Fry, D.L. (1969): Circ., 39, 40 (Suppl. 4), 38.
(12) Fry, D.L. (1973): In Atherogenesis: Initiating Factors. Ciba Foundation Symposium 12: Elsevier, 93.
(13) Caro, C.G., Fitz-Gerald, J.M. and Schroter, R.C. (1969): Nature, 223, 1159.
(14) Caro, C.G., Fitz-Gerald, J.M. and Schroter, R.C. (1971): Proc. Roy. Soc. Lond. (Biol.), 177, 109.
(15) Caro, C.G. (1973): In Atherogenesis: Initiating Factors. Ciba Foundation Symposium 12: Elsevier, 127.
(16) Bergel, D.H., Nerem, R.M. and Schwartz, C.J. (1976): Atherosclerosis, 23, 253.
(17) Day, A.J., Bell, F.P. and Schwartz, C.J. (1974): Exp. Molec. Pathol., 21, 179.
(18) Bell, F.P., Day, A.J., Gent, M. and Schwartz, C.J. (1975): Exp. Molec. Pathol., 22, 366.
(19) Bell, F.P., Adamson I.L. and Schwartz, C.J. (1974): Exp. Molec. Pathol., 20, 57.
(20) Bell, F.P., Gallus, A.S. and Schwartz, C.J. (1974): Exp. Molec. Pathol., 20, 281.
(21) Smith, E.B., Slater, R.S. and Hunter, J.A. (1973): Atherosclerosis, 18, 479.
(22) Smith, E.B. (1977): Amer. J. Pathol., 86, 665.
(23) Duguid, J.B. (1948): J. Path. Bact., 60, 57.
(24) Woolf, N. and Crawford, T. (1960): J. Path. Bact., 80, 405.
(25) Kao, V.C. and Wissler, R.W. (1965): Exp. Molec. Pathol., 4, 465.
(26) Wyllie, J.C., More, R.H. and Haust, M.D. (1964): J. Path. Bact., 88, 335.
(27) Walton, K.W. and Williamson, N. (1968): J. Atheroscler. Res., 8, 599.
(28) Carstairs, K.C. (1965): J. Path. Bact., 90, 225.
(29) Stefanovich, V. and Gore, I. (1971): Exp. Molec. Pathol., 14, 20.
(30) Gerrity, R.G. and Schwartz, C.J. (1977): Endothelial cell injury in early mild hypercholesterolemia. In Progress in Biochemical Pharmacology. Proceedings of the First International Atherosclerosis Conference, Vienna, 1977. Karger, Switzerland. (In press).
(31) Luft, J.H. (1966): Fed. Proc., 25, 1773.
(32) Gerrity, R.G., Richardson, M., Somer, J.B., Bell, F.P. and Schwartz, C.J.

(1977): Endothelial cell morphology in areas of in vivo Evans Blue uptake in the young pig aorta. II. Ultrastructure of the intima in areas of differing permeability to proteins. Amer. J. Pathol. (In press).

(33) Gerrity, R.G. and Schwartz, C.J. (1977): Structural correlates of arterial endothelial permeability in the Evans Blue Model. In Progress in Biochemical Pharmacology. Proceedings of the First International Atherosclerosis Conference, Vienna, 1977. Karger, Switzerland. (In press).

(34) Caplan, B.A. and Schwartz, C.J. (1973): Atherosclerosis, 17, 401.

(35) Caplan, B.A., Gerrity, R.G. and Schwartz, C.J. (1974): Exp. Molec. Pathol., 21, 102.

(36) Day, A.J. and Wahlqvist, M.L. (1968): Circ. Res., 23, 779.

(37) Geer, J.C. and Guidry, M.A. (1964): Exp. Molec. Pathol., 3, 485.

(38) Dayton, S. and Hashimoto, S. (1970): Exp. Molec. Pathol., 13, 253.

(39) Somer, J.B. and Schwartz, C.J. (1974): Atherosclerosis, 20, 507.

(40) Somer, J.B., Bell, F.P. and Schwartz, C.J. (1974): Atherosclerosis, 20, 11.

(41) Somer, J.B., Gerrity, R.G. and Schwartz, C.J. (1976): Exp. Molec. Pathol., 24, 1.

(42) Somer, J.B. and Schwartz, C.J. (1976): Exp. Molec. Pathol., 24, 129.

(43) Morrison, A.D., Berwick, L., Orci, L. and Winegrad, A.L. (1976): J. Clin. Invest., 57, 650.

(44) Gerrity, R.G., Richardson, M., Caplan, B.A., Cade, J., Hirsh, J. and Schwartz, C.J. (1976): Exp. Molec. Pathol., 24, 59.

(45) Schwartz, C.J. and Mitchell, J.R.A. (1962): Circ. Res., 11, 63.

(46) Mitchell, J.R.A. and Schwartz, C.J. (1965): In Arterial Disease. Blackwell Scientific Publications, Oxford.

(47) Ross, R. and Glomset, J. (1976): N. Engl. J. Med., 295, 369, 420.

(48) Ross, R., Glomset, J. and Harker, L. (1977): Amer. J. Pathol., 86, 675.

(49) Gospodarowicz, D., Moran, J., Braun, D. and Birdwell, C. (1976): Proc. Natl. Acad. Sci., 73, 4120.

(50) Gospodarowicz, D. and Moran, J.S. (1976): Ann. Rev. Biochem., 45, 531.

(51) Jimenez De Asua, L., Clingan, D. and Rudland, P.S. (1975): Proc. Natl. Acad. Sci., 72, 2724.

(52) Fischer-Dzoga, K., Fraser, R. and Wissler, R.W. (1976): Exp. Molec. Pathol., 24, 346.

(53) Fischer-Dzoga, K. and Wissler, R.W. (1976): Atherosclerosis, 24, 515.

(54) Benditt, E.P. and Benditt, J.M. (1973): Proc. Natl. Acad. Sci., 70, 1753.

(55) Benditt, E.P. (1977): Amer. J. Pathol., 86, 693.

(56) Pearson, T.A., Wang, A., Solez, K. and Heptinstall, R.H. (1975): Amer. J. Pathol., 81, 379.

(57) Peters, T.J., Takano, T. and DeDuve, C. (1973): In Atherogenesis: Initiating Factors. Ciba Foundation Symposium 12: 197.

(58) Brown, M.S. and Goldstein, J.L. (1976): Science, 191, 150.

(59) Brown, M.S. and Goldstein, J.L. (1975): Naturwissenschaften, 62, 385.

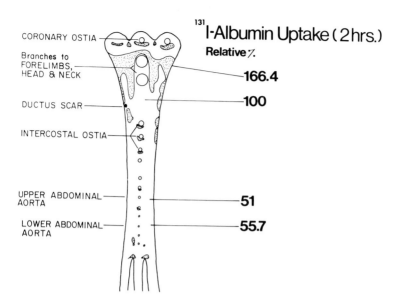

FIG. 2 ^{131}I-albumin uptake in the pig aorta 2 hours after injection of the labelled albumin. Stippled areas represent areas of Evans Blue dye uptake. Uptake is expressed as relative percentage, taking uptake in thoracic white areas as 100%.

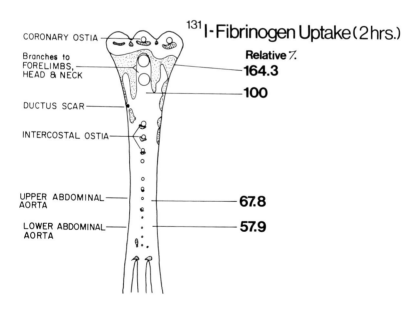

FIG. 3 ^{131}I-fibrinogen uptake in the pig aorta 2 hours after injection of the labelled fibrinogen. Data is expressed as in Fig. 2.

56

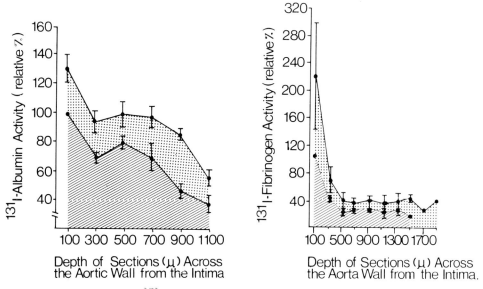

FIG. 4 Distribution of ^{131}I-albumin activity across the aortic wall is blue (upper) and white (lower) areas from the aortic arch 2 hours after administration of the isotope. The intimal surface is to the left and, the outer media to the right.

FIG. 5 Distribution of ^{131}I-fibrinogen activity across the aortic wall in blue (upper) and white (lower) areas of the thoracic aorta 2 hours after intravenous injection of the isotope. The intimal surface is to the left, and the outer media to the right.

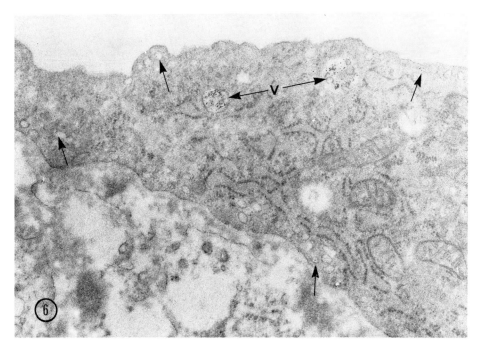

FIG. 6 Transmission electron micrograph of endothelium from a blue area in the pig aortic arch five minutes after ferritin injection. Ferritin (seen as black dots) is found in pinocytotic vesicles (arrows) and concentrated in larger multivesicular vacuoles (V). Unstained section X47,500.

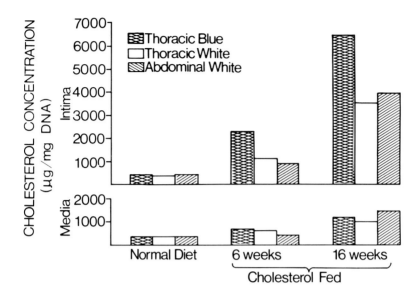

FIG. 7   Schematic diagram depicting pinocytotic uptake and transport of extracellular macromolecules by endothelial cells. Vesicles containing macromolecules bud off the plasma membrane and pass into the cytoplasm. Con-
tents may be released inside the cell and utilized, or released on to the
extracellular space on another cellular surface. Transendothelial vesicular transport may be bi-directional.

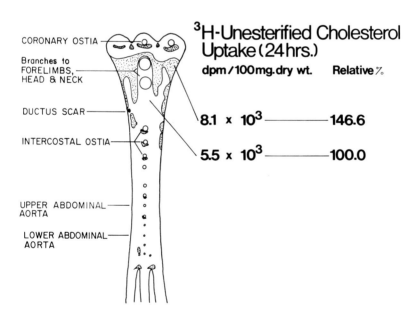

FIG. 8   The cholesterol concentration (ug/mg DNA) in blue and white areas of the
aortic intima and media of pigs on a normal diet, or receiving cholesterol-
containing diets for 6 or 16 weeks.

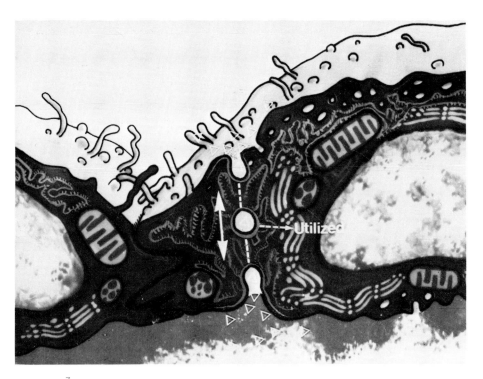

FIG. 9 ^{3}H-unesterified cholesterol uptake in blue (stippled) and white (plain) areas in the thoracic aorta of the young healthy pig 24 hours after administration of the isotope cholesterol. Results are expressed both as dpm and relative percentages.

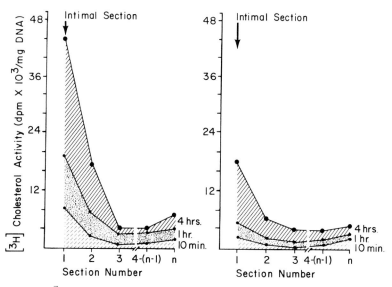

FIG. 10 ^{3}H-cholesterol transmural aortic gradients in blue (left panel) and white (right panel) areas, 10 minutes, 1 hour, and 4 hours after injection of the isotope. The intimal surface of the aorta is arrowed. Activity at each level across the aorta is expressed as dpm x 10^3/mg DNA.

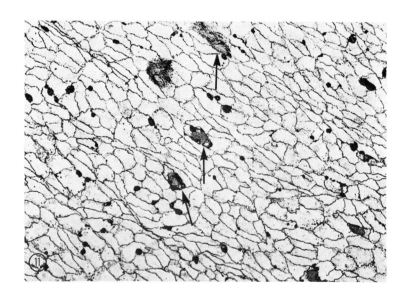

FIG. 11 Silver nitrate-stained Hautchen preparation of aortic endothelium from a
         blue area. Endothelial cell boundaries are stained, giving "pavement-like"
         appearance. Dead or injured endothelial cells show intense uptake of
         silver stain (arrows). X900.

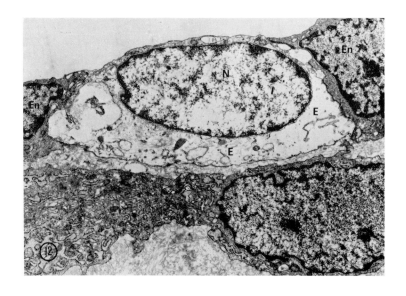

FIG. 12 Transmission electron micrographs of a dead endothelial cell (E), with
         normal endothelial cells (En) on either side. Cytoplasm is watery and
         vacuolated (V). Nucleus (N) shows dispersion of chromatin and appears
         smaller. X11,500.

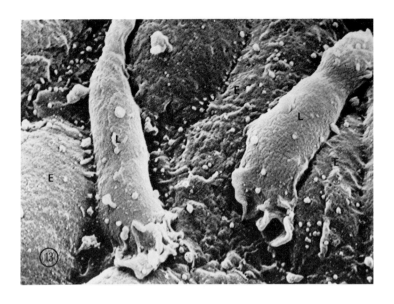

FIG. 13   Scanning electron micrograph from a blue area in the aortic arch of a pig
fed a lard-cholesterol diet for four weeks.   Two leukocytes (L) are adherent to the underlying endothelium (E).   X13,500.

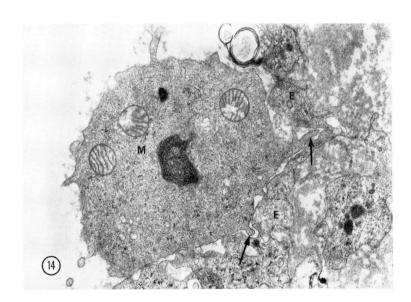

FIG. 14   Transmission electron micrograph of a monocyte (M) adherent to white area
endothelium (E) from a pig fed lard-cholesterol diet for two weeks.   Note
pseudopods (arrows) from monocyte extending into the endothelium.   X21,900.

EXERCISE, STRESS OR WHAT? THE NON-INVASIVE DETECTION OF LATENT CORONARY ARTERY
DISEASE

John Coltart

St. Thomas's Hospital, London

Coronary artery disease has assumed epidemic proportions in many countries of the
world where it causes between one third to one half of all deaths. There is a wide
spectrum of presentation of patients with coronary artery disease. This communication will discuss the methods of detecting latent coronary artery disease in an
entirely asymptomatic individual with no previous symptoms or signs suggestive of
coronary artery disease.

Table 1 outlines the methods of detecting coronary artery disease. Clearly post-
mortem analysis of the heart is of little value in the quest to prevent the problem
of coronary artery disease. Coronary angiography is a highly invasive procedure
and cannot be employed as a screening procedure for latent coronary artery disease.
This presentation is directed to discuss the non-invasive detection of latent
coronary artery disease in the hope that some therapy may be instituted to prevent
or retard the clinical manifestation and the problems resulting from coronary artery
disease.

TABLE 1

METHODS		DIAGNOSIS
1.	History and clinical examination	
2.	Family history	
3.	Risk factors	
4.	Resting E.C.G.	
5.	Ambulatory E.C.G. monitoring	Myocardial
6.	Stress exercise monitoring	Ischaemia
7.	Echocardiography	
8.	Isotope scanning	Coronary
9.	Coronary angiography	Artery Disease
10.	Post mortem	

EXERCISE STRESS TESTING

The resting and ambulatory electrocardiogram are relatively poor predictors of the
presence of significant coronary artery disease or the possibility of future
'Coronary Target Events'. Since manifestations of coronary artery disease are
generally best provoked under conditions of stress various methods have been produced to stress the subject and thus to reveal evidence of coronary artery disease
not obvious at rest. For a relatively uncomplicated outpatient assessment, the use
of exercise is now widely established and the relevance of the findings thus provoked is well understood in relation to symptomatic coronary artery disease if less
so in the asymptomatic population.

For any diagnostic test it is important to be aware of the influence of the prevalence of a disease process on the significance of a positive result in the test; and to consider certain definitions in the interpretation of such tests.

DEFINITIONS:

SENSITIVITY: Percentage of times the test is abnormal in a subgroup with the disease process.

SPECIFICITY: Percentage of times the test is normal in a subgroup without the disease process.

RELATIVE
RISK: Likelihood of disease in those with positive test compared with those with negative test.

PREDICTIVE
VALUE OF
ABNORMAL
TEST: Percentage of those with abnormal test who have disease.

FALSE
POSITIVE
RATE: 100 - Predictive value (percent)

DERIVATIONS:

$$\text{SENSITIVITY} = \frac{TP}{TP + FN} \times 100$$

$$\text{RELATIVE RISK} = \frac{TP}{TP + FP} \bigg/ \frac{FN}{TN + FN}$$

$$\text{SPECIFICITY} = \frac{TN}{FP + TN} \times 100$$

$$\text{PREDICTIVE VALUE} = \frac{TP}{TP + FP} \times 100$$

TP (True positive). Abnormal test and disease.

FN (False negative). Normal test and disease.

TN (True negative). Normal test. No disease.

FP (False positive). Abnormal test. No disease.

Redwood, Borer and Epstein (1), have emphasised the influence of disease prevalence on the predictive accuracy of a positive exercise test. Thus, assuming a sensitivity 95% and specificity 95% for any diagnostic test, if the disease prevalence is 90%, the predictive accuracy is 99%; if the disease prevalence is 2%, the predictive accuracy is 28%. Hence as prevalence diminishes the number of false positive tests increases. In the case of coronary artery disease in a selected hospital population referred for evaluation of chest pain the prevalence of coronary artery disease is approximately 90%. In an unselected asymptomatic population (depending on age) the prevalence of coronary artery disease is 1 to 5%. In general, exercise testing has an overall sensitivity of approximately 70% and specificity 90%.

METHODS OF STRESS TESTING

1.   Single load exercise test 'two step' (2)
                              'double two step'

2. Graded exercise test Bicycle ergometer
                              Treadmill

3. Isometric Hand Grip

4. Hypoxaemia

5. Atrial pacing

6. Isoprenaline infusion

The single load stress test is adversely influenced by the considerable variation in exercise tolerance between patients because of the difference in degree of coronary artery disease and level of physical training. Graded exercise testing allows improved sensitivity, this is well reviewed by Redwood and Epstein (3). In a comparative study of 30 patients with angina pectoris the sensitivity of multi-stage exercise testing was 80% and Masters' two step test 57% (4).

In all testing programmes it is important to have a defined protocol such as that for progressive treadmill exercise produced by Bruce and his colleagues, (5) and definite end points to exercise. The commonly employed end points consist of:

1. Angina

2. ST segment depression equal or greater than 1 mm (100 uV) which is horizontal or downsloping from the ST junction persisting for 0.08 secs. after end of QRS complex, the abnormality should be present in 3 consecutive beats during exercise or in the initial 3 minutes of recovery after exercise.

3. Complex ventricular arrhythmias

    i.   Coupled ventricular premature beats (VPB)

    ii. Frequent VPB

    iii. Multiform VPB

    iv. R on T phenomenon

    v.   Ventricular tachycardia

4. Breathlessness

5. Fatigue or ataxia

6. Target heart rate (85 - 90% of predicted maximum heart rate for age and sex).

In general less than 5% will fail to achieve end points 1,2,3, or 6. During exercise the following should be monitored:

1. Work capacity   Total work performed
                   Time into exercise protocol

2. Heart rate

3. Blood pressure

4. ST changes

5. Arrhythmias

ST segment changes are well documented as occurring during spontaneous or exercise induced angina. Myocardial lactate monitoring studies have shown abnormal myocardial lactate metabolism developing at the time of diminution of LV function indices and ST segment changes, all of which precede the development of angina. There is good evidence to suggest that ST segment changes are a reflection of myocardial ischaemia at least in a proportion of cases. On both epidemiological grounds and coronary arteriographic grounds the appearance of ST changes on exercise are good predictors of future coronary events and of underlying obstructive coronary arterial disease in a symptomatic population (6 - 15).

1 mm (100 uV) of ST depression on exercise with a normal resting electrocardiogram is generally selected as a positive test result to optimise sensitivity and specificity of the test. ST elevation is seen in some exercise studies - in leads with Q waves this probably represents LV asynergy - in other situations it may represent the variant form of angina as described by Prinzmetal and probably due in the majority of cases to coronary arterial spasm. There is an inverse relationship between sensitivity and specificity when different ST criteria are selected in that the greater the ST depression considered to represent a positive response (0.5 mm/1 mm/ 2 mms) the greater the specificity of the test but the lower the sensitivity. Thus Mason (7) in a study of 84 patients with coronary artery anatomy documented at arteriography used these criteria for ST depression:

ST depression	Sensitivity	Specificity
0.5 mm	88%	69%
1.0 mm	84%	83%
2.0 mm	78%	89%

Overall for the employment of 2.0 mm ST depression instead of 1.0 mm ST depression for a positive test result in patients with symptomatic coronary artery disease, the sensitivity of the exercise stress test is reduced from 70% to 50% with a gain of specificity and an enhancement of predictive accuracy. Table 2 summarises the correlation of an abnormal stress test defined as 1 mm or greater ST depression on exercise (or during recovery) with documented significant coronary artery disease (greater than 50% stenosis) in patients with symptoms suggestive of ischaemic heart disease (7 - 15).

TABLE 2

			n	Sensitivity %	Specificity %
(7)	Mason	1967	84	78	89
(8)	Kassebaum	1968	68	71	97
(9)	Roitman	1970	46	80	88
(10)	Ascoop	1971	96	59	94
(11)	Martin	1972	100	62	89
(12)	Keleman	1973	74	54	96
(13)	Bartel	1974	650	65	92
(14)	Froelicher	1976	52	77	73
(15)	Goldshlager	1976	410	64	93
	Total		1580 mean	68	90

Enhancement of sensitivity may be achieved by more strict criteria of ST depression, by the use of multiple ECG leads, by further analysis of the ST segment by computer analytical techniques or by serial exercise testing.

The most commonly employed ECG monitoring lead is V5 or a bipolar derivative such as CB5 or CM5. These will detect most of the ST segment abnormalities occurring during or after exercise testing (V5 89%) (16).

However, in 10 to 20% of positive exercise ECG tests these ST segment changes will
be detected only in leads other than V5. Mason found 19/56 positive tests showing
ST changes in one lead only, 17 of which were other than V5. Phibbs and Buckels
(17) in a study of 947 patients employing 12 lead ECG monitoring found 147 positive
tests of which 38 were positive only in leads other than V5 (21.1%). (See Table 3).

TABLE 3

	n	%
II, III, aVF	23	12.8
II, III, aVF, V6	3	1.6
V6	5	2.8
V4	3	1.7
V1	1	0.55
I	1	0.55
V2, V3, V4	2	1.1
	38	21.1

This may account for some of the false negative tests in studies employing single
lead systems only. Further analysis of the ST segment with respect to ST slope
in those tests with junctional ST depression and upsloping ST segments, or area
between ST segment and isoelectric line (SX Integral) together with computer analysis to reduce observer error may improve sensitivity and specificity as described
by Ascoop (18). Serial exercise testing may also usefully improve the sensitivity
of testing. In one such series without arteriographic confirmation of coronary
artery disease, Doyle followed 2,003 subjects with no history of angina or previous
infarction and a negative exercise test on admission to the study. Of 75 patients
developing a positive stress test during the study, 85% developed overt coronary
artery disease over a 5 year follow-up period (in 30% of 264 patients developing
overt coronary artery disease conversion of the test was the first indication of
coronary artery disease) while of those remaining negative the incidence of overt
coronary artery disease over a 5 year period was 1.5% (19). This latter is an
example of the potential value of exercise testing in defining a group of asymptomatic individuals with a higher than normal risk of subsequent coronary events. In
four other studies of exercise testing in asymptomatic individuals, the sensitivity,
specificity, predictive accuracy and relative risks of the development of clinically
apparent coronary artery disease, are outlined in Table 4.

TABLE 4

			n	+ve	Cor.events	ST crit.	sens	spec	Pred. acc.	Risk ratio
(20)	Bruce	1969	221	10%	2.3% 5 yr	1 mm	60	91	13.6	13.6x
(21)	Aronow	1975	100	13%	9% 5 yr	1 mm	66	92	46	13.6x
(22)	Froelicher	1974	451	3.8%	3.8% 6.3 yr	1 mm	59	94	26	15.1x
(23)	Cumming	1975	510	12%	5.1% 3 yr	2 mm	58	91	25	10x

n: number, +ve: positive tests, Cor. events: percentage of patient population
subsequently manifesting coronary diseases.

Overall predictive accuracy is approximately 25% and the prevalence of coronary
artery disease averages 4.4%, confirming the limiting effect of low prevalence of
disease on the value of a positive test result.

Relatively few studies have been performed on asymptomatic individuals where a
positive test has been followed by coronary arteriography, three studies are listed
in Table 5.

TABLE 5

		n	CAD 75%+	any CAD	N.C.A.
			POSITIVE EXERCISE TESTS		
(24)	Froelicher Aircrew	111	34 (34%)	51 (46%)	60 (54%)
(25)	Borer Lipid clinic	30	11 (37%)	20 (67%)	10 (33%)
(26)	Erikssen Factory workers in Norway	88	58 (66%)	-	30 (34%)

These results of which the study of Erikssen in Norwegian factory workers is perhaps
the only unselected asymptomatic group suggest that a positive exercise test is
falsely positive in a large number of such individuals confirming the low predictive
accuracy in populations with a low prevalence of coronary artery disease.

Exercise induced ventricular arrhythmias do not in general have the malign prognostic
value that was once believed. In fact, 50% of normal individuals will display some
ventricular premature beats of heart rates 150 to 170 per minute - they are probably
more common in individuals with coronary artery disease but are a poor predictor of
obstructive disease or subsequent cardiac events. Froelicher, using a frequency of
ventricular premature beats of greater than 1/5 or 3 or more ventricular premature
beats consecutively during exercise testing found over a 6.3 year follow-up a sensitivity of 6.5%, predictive value 10.3% and relative risk of coronary target events
of 3.4x although association with ST changes strongly suggested extensive underlying
coronary artery disease (22).

The duration of exercise is an important predictor of prognosis in patients with
known coronary artery disease as discussed by Bruce in this symposium. The combination of limited exercise duration (less than 3 minutes), peak systolic blood pressure less than 130 Hg and cardiomegaly on a chest X ray carries a very high yearly
mortality 880/1000 (1 factor present 95/1000, 2 factors present 250/1000).

Careful attention to technical detail in elimination of false positive tests and
awareness of physiological and pathological causes of false positive tests are important in the interpretation of the results of exercise stress testing, some of
these factors are listed in Table 6.

TABLE 6

Possible causes of false positive test:

Factors affecting interpretation of ST response to exercise

       Incorrect ST criteria

       Sudden excessive stress

       Inadequate recording equipment

       Improper lead system

       Position post-exercise

       Time pattern of ST depression

Abnormal ST depression without coronary artery disease

       Valvular HD

       Congenital HD

       Cardiomyopathies

       Pericardial disease

       Drugs - Digitalis

       Electrolyte abnormalities

       Non-fasting state

       Anaemia

       Hyperventilation

       Hypertension

       Wolff-Parkinson-White syndrome

       Mitral leaflet prolapse syndrome

       Vasoregulatory abnormalities

       Left ventricular hypertrophy with strain

       Bundle branch block

The role of exercise electrocardiography in the detection of a group of subjects with severe coronary artery disease has recently been studied by Goldschlager et al. (15). The ST response to exercise was categorised into 4 groups, IA and IB being the classical 'ischaemic' response IA, down-sloping and IB horizontal ST segment depression and II junctional ST depression with upsloping ST segment.

For 410 subjects with varying likelihood of coronary artery disease the results were as follows:

TABLE 7

| Type I response | | Sensitivity 64% | | Specificity 93% (n = 330) | |
| Type I + II response | | Sensitivity 76% | | Specificity 82% | |

| | | Normal | Number of coronary arteries with 50% or greater disease | | |
ST response	n	coronary artery	I	II	III
IA	123	0.8%	9%	34%	56%
IB	60	15%	27%	20%	38%
II	47	32%	13%	21%	32%
Negative	180	65%	20%	12%	3%

Thus the use of Type II response increases the sensitivity of the test but with loss of specificity.

Isolated left anterior descending disease or 'left main stem equivalent' lesions did not produce a specific response on exercise testing allowing prediction. From this and other studies certain pointers to more severe (triple vessel and left main) coronary artery disease may be determined, these include the type IA response during exercise especially occurring early in the exercise protocol and of long duration during the recovery phase; a marked depth of ST depression ($>$ 2 mms), complex ventricular arrhythmias and hypotension also are suggestive. However, it should not be forgotten that severe coronary artery disease may be associated with a normal exercise test (27).

To summarise the use of exercise E.C.G. testing. In an epidemiological sense this test is valuable in defining groups of symptomatic or asymptomatic individuals who have a high risk of subsequent 'target coronary events' although what to do with this information remains controversial. In a diagnostic situation the ECG response to exercise is a good predictor of underlying coronary artery disease in a population with symptoms (high prevalence coronary artery disease) although it adds little to a carefully taken history (sensitivity 84%, specificity 75%) (10) except to define a group of patients with a significant risk of severe proximal disease - but since this group has a high risk of myocardial infarction and are generally good candidates for surgery this is an important application. In an asymptomatic population (low prevalence coronary artery disease) the incidence of false positive responses is high and predictive accuracy low so its diagnostic use in this situation must inevitably be limited.

ECHOCARDIOGRAPHY
The use of ultrasound as a diagnostic aid was introduced into clinical medicine by Edler and Hertz in 1953. Initial application of the technique was to detect valvular abnormalities but with increasing experience and refinement of instrumentation it is now widely applied to the study of overall and regional left ventricular function. In the experimental situation hypokinesia or akinesia of the left ventricular myocardium rapidly follows partial or complete occlusion of the coronary artery supplying that region of myocardium. In the clinical situation, despite being complicated by the slowly progressive nature of the reduction in coronary arterial blood flow and the opportunity for the development of a collateral circulation, left ventricular regional dysfunction is commonly demonstrated by contrast cineangiography in the presence of obstructive coronary arterial disease even in the absence of myocardial infarction. Following stress, exaggerating the imbalance of myocardial oxygen supply and demand, (atrial pacing, isoprenaline infusion or exercise) such regional dysfunction may be exaggerated or precipitated. Reversibility of

70

regional dysfunction in the presence of myocardial ischaemia is demonstrated after the above provocation tests by the administration of glyceryl trinitrate and, in some instances, by improvement following successful vein-graft surgery. Obstructive coronary arterial disease is the major cause of regional myocardial dysfunction.

Echocardiography can be used to define left ventricular cavity dimensions and the muscle thickness and excursion of the left ventricular walls. Employing the M-mode echocardiographic 'sweep' from the region of the mitral valve towards the apex much of the interventricular septum and the posterior left ventricular wall can be visualised and the excursion of these two regions of myocardium studied. Infarction, fibrosis and ischaemia (acute or chronic) will lead to a reduction of amplitude of excursion and in some instances to frankly paradoxical movement. Exaggerated normal movement of the left ventricular wall suggests compensation for a region of abnormal function elsewhere. Normal septal excursion is greater than 3 mms; normal posterior LV wall excursion is greater than 8 mms (1, 2). Reduced septal excursion is a good predictor of the presence of significant left anterior descending coronary artery disease (sensitivity 80%, specificity 69%) and reduced posterior LV wall movement a reasonable predictor of left circumflex disease (left dominant system) or right coronary artery disease (right dominant system), (sensitivity 52%, specificity 67%) in patients with stable angina pectoris studied at rest in the absence of previous myocardial infarction (1). Correlation of left ventricular (LV) cineangiography and echocardiography is good (2). Of 38 patients with significant coronary artery disease, 25 demonstrated left ventricular asynergy - 24 with abnormal wall movement on echocardiography - 8 patients had normal left ventricular angiography and abnormal echocardiography - 5 patients had normal LV angiography and echocardiography. To some extent the false positive echocardiographic trace may represent the true situation in that different parts of the LV wall are viewed compared with single or biplane cineangiography and the septum represents a region which is difficult to evaluate on cineangiography. Correlation with previous evidence of transmural myocardial infarction (Q waves in the resting ECG) are excellent; in 20 such patients, 18 demonstrated echocardiographic wall movement abnormality in the predicted area of infarction, one showed abnormal septal movement with previous inferior infarction but with coexistent 90% stenosis of the left anterior descending artery and one showed exaggerated septal movement in the presence of anterior infarction due to left ventricular volume overload secondary to mitral regurgitation (2). Demonstration of reversible abnormality of septal movement has been shown in the presence of high grade proximal left anterior descending coronary artery stenosis (2), and with variant angina due to anterior descending coronary arterial spasm (3), both precipitated by isometric hand-grip exercise during echocardiographic recording. Attempts to correlate septal movement abnormalities with anterior descending coronary arterial disease proximal or distal to the first septal perforating branch have not proved sufficiently accurate to be clinically useful (4).

The foregoing describes the situation in populations with a high prevalence of coronary artery disease, whether these techniques will prove useful in asymptomatic populations remains to be evaluated.

Cross-sectional echocardiography has been recently demonstrated to visualise the left main coronary artery with considerable consistency, demonstrating significant obstruction of the lumen of this vessel in selected cases (5). This is clearly an important advance in the diagnosis of this high risk group when such patients are asymptomatic.

ISOTOPE TECHNIQUES
Isotope techniques are being increasingly employed in the detection and assessment of coronary artery disease in that they may enable the confirmation of the presence of ischaemia, the extent and location of the underlying coronary artery disease and the effect of ischaemia on overall and regional left ventricular function.

Three groups of techniques are commonly employed:

1.   Assessment of myocardial perfusion.

2.   Labelling of acute myocardial infarction.

3.   Overall and regional left ventricular function studies.

Myocardial perfusion studies generally employ monovalent cations which can be administered intravenously at rest or during exercise. Tissue uptake (particularly myocardial uptake) is proportional to blood flow at the time of administration of the isotope and areas of reduced myocardial perfusion will be visualised on subsequent gamma-camera scans as 'cold' areas. Studies at rest will show resting ischaemia or previous infarction and the development of new perfusion defects, compared with the resting scan, when the isotope is administered during exercise suggest significant myocardial ischaemia with underlying coronary artery disease in the majority of cases.

Isotopes of Potassium were initially studied and K^{43} despite technical problems with imaging has proved a useful agent in that over a range of coronary flow rates from normal to severely reduced flow, myocardial uptake parallels myocardial blood flow. Zaret et al. (1973) have shown normal resting and exercise K^{43} myocardial perfusion scans in 9 patients with false positive exercise ECG tests in the presence of documented normal coronary arteriograms (1). The specificity of exercise ECG testing may thus be considerably improved.

Thallium 201 was originally suggested as an isotope for myocardial perfusion imaging by Kanawa in 1970 and used experimentally by Lebowitz in 1973. The physical half life is approximately 72 hours. Tissue uptake is flow determined, 70% of the isotope being removed by a single passage through the myocardium resulting in rapid blood clearance and development of a stable myocardial image. The myocardial half life is 7 to 24 hours, there is slow washout of the isotope and subsequent redistribution so that eventual distribution reflects potassium space. Myocardial Thallium 201 distribution has been shown to closely follow myocardial regional perfusion, using simultaneously administered labelled microspheres as a measure of perfusion in complete and partial coronary artery occlusion (2, 3). In the clinical situation studying patients with symptoms suggestive of ischaemic heart disease or evidence of previous myocardial infarction (a population with very high prevalence of coronary artery disease) the test has been shown to be reproducible in that injections of Thallium 201 at the peak of identical maximal exercise tests produced identical segmental perfusion patterns in 64 of 70 myocardial segments studied in 14 patients (4), while lower levels of exercise produced a considerably lower yield of perfusion abnormalities compared with maximal exercise.

Comparison of rest and exercise Thallium 201 myocardial perfusion scans with rest and exercise ECG and with coronary artery anatomy shows good correlation for evidence of previous myocardial infarction with a defect on the rest Thallium scan, Q waves on the rest ECG, left ventricular hypokinesia on left ventricular cineangiography and significant disease in the supplying coronary artery (5, 6). Perfusion defects in excess of those predicted by the presence of previous myocardial infarctions are seen on the rest scan also in territories with severe underlying coronary artery disease suggesting reduced myocardial perfusion at rest. Resting perfusion in an individual with normal coronary arteries may be somewhat patchy but apart from an area of diminished Thallium uptake at the apex, frequently noted, false positive rest scans are rare. After exercise, perfusion in normal individuals is greatly increased and relatively uniform, perfusion defects present at rest are generally similar or more prominent and new perfusion defects are noted in territories with significant underlying coronary artery disease but without evidence of infarction. There is a tendency for increasing numbers of defects with increasing extent and severity of coronary artery disease (5). Compared with the exercise ECG, Thallium scanning on exercise is considerably more sensitive although most of this difference resides in the number in whom the exercise ECG is uninterpretable due to previous infarctions, conduction defects and arrhythmias and in the number failing to achieve near maximal predicted heart rate on exercise (5). There should be no false positive Thallium perfusion scans on exercise but there is an incidence of patients negative on both Thallium scanning and exercise ECG despite significant underlying coronary artery disease (7).

In a recent study of segmental perfusion using Thallium 201 administered at rest and during exercise Lenaers and his colleagues (1977) have shown observer disagreement of 7.5% and using segments other than the apical segment good ability to demonstrate significant disease (greater than 50% stenosis) in left anterior descending coronary artery (sensitivity 84%, specificity 95%), right coronary artery (sensitivity 79%, specificity 88%) and to a lesser extent left circumflex coronary artery (sensitivity 49%, specificity 89%). Good discrimination was obtained in prediction of single vessel disease and multiple vessel disease and the overall detection of coronary artery disease was excellent (sensitivity 95%, specificity 93%, false negative 18%, false positive 2% (a single patient with isolated 50% stenosis of the left circumflex coronary artery)). The high sensitivity in this study is related to the selected population and the inclusion of defects present on both rest and exercise scans.

To avoid repeated administration of isotope it has been suggested that administration of Thallium at peak exercise with repeat scanning over the subsequent hours will allow distinction of ischaemia and infarction. A defect representing infarction should remain unaltered while redistribution of isotope after exercise should result in gradual infilling of defects due to ischaemia. This has been verified experimentally and also in a limited series of patients with ischaemia or myocardial infarction (8).

In summary myocardial perfusion imaging should enhance the sensitivity and specificity of exercise testing in the symptomatic population and should also be helpful in the asymptomatic population although data on such populations is as yet extremely limited.

Acute infarct labelling has little relevance to the very early detection of coronary artery disease.

Assessment of overall and regional left ventricular function using gated blood pool scanning at rest and possibly also during exercise has potentially very wide applications in ischaemic heart disease and in combination with myocardial perfusion scanning in the assessment of symptomatic ischaemic heart disease and the detection of ischaemia and coronary artery disease in the asymptomatic population.

REFERENCES

EXERCISE STRESS TESTING
(1) Redwood, D.R., Borer, J.S. and Epstein, S.E. (1976): Circulation, 54, 703.
(2) Master, A.M. and Oppenheimer, E.T. (1929): American Journal of Medical Science, 177, 223.
(3) Redwood, D.R. and Epstein, S.E. (1972): Circulation, 46, 1115.
(4) Mason, R.E. and Likar, I. (1964): Transactions of the American Clinical and Climatological Association, 76, 40.
(5) Bruce, R.A., Blackman, J.R., Jones, J.W. and Swait, G. (1963): Paediatrics, 32, Suppl. 4, 742.
(6) Robb, G.P. and Marks, H.H. (1967): J.A.M.A., 200, 918.
(7) Mason, R.E., Likar, I., Biern, R.O. and Ross, R.S. (1967): Circulation, 36, 517.
(8) Kassebaum, D.G., Sutherland, K.I. and Judkins, M.P. (1968): American Heart Journal, 75, 759.
(9) Roitman, D., Jones, W.B. and Sheffield, L.T. (1970): Annals of Internal Medi-

cine, 72, 641.

(10) Ascoop, C.A., Simoons, M.L., Egmond, W.G. and Bruschke, A.V.G. (1971): American Heart Journal, 82, 609.

(11) Martin, C.M. and McConahay, D.R. (1972): Circulation, 46, 956.

(12) Kelemen, M.H., Gillilan, R.E., Bouchard, R.J., Heppner, R.L. and Warbasse, J.R. (1973): Circulation, 48, 1227.

(13) Bartel, A.G., Behar, V.S., Peter, R.H., Orgain, E.S. and Kong, Y. (1974): Circulation, 49, 348.

(14) Froelicher, V.F., Thompson, A.J., Longo, M.R., Triebwasser, J.H. and Lancaster, M.C. (1976): Progress in Cardiovascular Disease, 18, 265.

(15) Goldschlager, N., Selzer, A. and Cohn, K. (1976): Annals of Internal Medicine, 85, 277.

(16) Blackburn, H., Taylor, H.L., Okamoto, N., Mitchell, P.L., Rautaharju, P.M., Mitchell, P.L. and Kerkhof, A.C. (1967): In 'Physical Activity and the Heart'. Ed. Karvonen, M. and Barry, A. Springfield, Illinois. Charles C. Thomas.

(17) Phibbs, B.P. and Buckels, L.J. (1975): American Heart Journal, 90, 275.

(18) Ascoop, C.A., Distelbrink, C.A. and de Lang, P.A. (1977): British Heart Journal, 39, 212.

(19) Doyle, J.T. and Kinch, S.H. (1970): Circulation, 41, 545.

(20) Bruce, R.A. and McDonough, J.R. (1969): Bulletin of New York Academy of Medicine, 45, 1288.

(21) Aronow, W.S. and Cassidy, J. (1975): Circulation, 52, 616.

(22) Froelicher, V.F., Thomas, M.M., Pillow, C. and Lancaster, M.C. (1974): American Journal of Cardiology, 34, 770.

(23) Cumming, G.R., Samm, J., Borysyk, L. and Kich, L. (1975): Canadian Medical Association Journal, 112, 578.

(24) Froelicher, V.F., Yanowitz, F.G., Thompson, A.J. and Lancaster, M.C. (1973): Circulation, 48, 597.

(25) Borer, J.S., Brensike, J.F., Redwood, D.R., Itscoitz, S.B., Passamani, E.R., Stone, N.J., Richardson, J.M., Levy, R.I. and Epstein, S.E. (1975): New England Journal of Medicine, 293, 367.

(26) Erikssen, J., Enge, I., Forfang, K. and Storstein, O. (1976): Circulation, 54, 371.

(27) Bruce, R.A., Hornsten, T.R. and Blackmon, J.R. (1968): Circulation, 38, 552.

ISOTOPE TECHNIQUES

(1) Zaret, B.L., Stenson, R.E., Martin, N.D., Strauss, H.W., Wells, H.P., McGowan, R.L. and Flamm, M.D. (1973): Circulation, 48, 1234.

(2) Strauss, H.W., Harrison, K., Langan, J.K., Lebowitz, E. and Pitt, B. (1975): Circulation, 51, 641.

(3) Mueller, T.M., Marcus, M.L., Ehrhardt, J.C., Chaudhuri, T. and Abboud, F.M. (1976): Circulation, 54, 640.

(4) McLaughlin, P.R., Martin, R.P., Doherty, P., Daspit, S., Goris, M., Haskell, W., Lewis, S., Kriss, J.P. and Harrison, D.C. (1977): Circulation, 55, 497.

(5) Bailey, I.K., Griffith, L.S.C., Rouleau, J., Strauss, H.W. and Pitt, B. (1977): Circulation, 55, 79.

(6) Lenaers, A., Block, P., van Thiel, E., Lebedelle, M., Becquevort, P., Erbsmann, F. and Ermans, A.M. (1977): Journal of Nuclear Medicine, 18, 509.

(7) Pohost, G.M., Zir, L.M., Moore, R.H., McKusick, K.A., Guiney, T.E. and Beller, G.A. (1977): Circulation, 55, 294.

ECHOCARDIOGRAPHY

(1) Dortimer, A.C., DeJoseph, R.L., Shiroff, R.A., Liedtke, A.J. and Zelis, R. (1976): Circulation, 54, 724.

(2) Jacobs, J.J., Feigenbaum, H., Corya, B.C. and Phillips, J.F. (1973): Circulation, 48, 263.

(3) Widlansky, S., McHenry, P.L., Corya, B.C. and Phillips, J.F. (1975): American Heart Journal, 90, 631.

(4) Gordon, M.J. and Kerber, R.E. (1977): Circulation, 55, 338.

(5) Weyman, A.E., Feigenbaum, H., Dillon, J.C., Johnston, K.W. and Eggleton, R.C. (1976): Circulation, 54, 169.

MAXIMAL EXERCISE TESTING: A PRELIMINARY REPORT OF THE SEATTLE HEART WATCH[*]

Robert Bruce

Division of Cardiology, University of Washington, Seattle, Washington

INTRODUCTION

The value of exercise stress testing for early detection of coronary heart disease
is uncertain and controversial. Responsible factors include variations in purpose,
in criteria for selection and exclusion of individuals; and in methods, observations
and criteria for interpretation. Many studies have been directed towards evaluation of ST depression as an acute electrocardiographic manifestation of exertional
myocardial ischemia. Salient justifications for and limitations of this orientat-
ion are listed in Table 1. First is the association between ST depression and the
eventual clinical manifestations of coronary heart disease (1 - 6); next there is a
greater prevalence (7, 8) of ST depression when the severity of the exercise is increased, and there is evidence that ST depression can be elicited in both high (7)
and low-risk (8) population samples. There is also a greater sensitivity for detection of men at risk for subsequent coronary heart disease events when ST depression is elicited by maximal exercise testing (9, 10). Unfortunately the value of ST
depression is limited by observer variability and uncertainty about criteria (11),
and a high proportion of false-positive responses (12). Additional limitations of
this use of ST depression are listed in Table 2. ST depression is only a non-specific functional response to myocardial stress (13), and not equivalent to anatomical
evidence of coronary vascular or myocardial disease at rest. Many factors may contribute to this functional imbalance, which further limits its reliable application
in the presence of disease and associated therapy.

My purpose today is to present data reflecting a four-point study design (Table 3).
First, individuals were selected from both industrial and clinical populations.
Second, each was examined clinically at rest. Third, each was monitored during
exercise of progressive intensity to functional limits. Fourth, follow-up surveil-
ance for any subsequent manifestations of coronary heart disease events was conducted annually. The results represent only a preliminary report of studies that are
still in progress. They provide some insight into the value of exercise testing;
more important, they suggest the possibility for more efficient and cost-reducing
modifications of the study design for future applications.

MATERIAL

The material for this analysis was selected from two cohorts of the exercise testing unit of the Seattle Heart Watch. This was initiated in 1971 as a prospective
community study supported by the National Heart and Lung Institute. The numbers of
persons examined and tested, less those excluded, and differences in clinical manifestations in the absence of coronary heart disease are shown in Table 4. 1748 men
in an industrial cohort (tested at the Boeing Company's Medical Facility) and 1012
men in a clinical cohort (tested at a number of private offices, clinics and teach-
ing hospitals) were selected for this analysis. Of these, 2389 were healthy, asymptomatic men without apparent clinical manifestations of heart disease. 216 men were
classified as hypertensive without heart disease, and another 155 had atypical chest

[*] Supported by research contract and grant from the National Heart and Lung Institute
and grant from the Health Services Research Administration.

-pain syndromes without angina pectoris. The proportion of men with the hypertension or chest-pain syndromes ranged from 6.7 per cent in the industrial cohort to 25.2 per cent of those in the clinical cohort.

These differences reflect selective processes with respect to health standards for employment, diverse reasons for being examined and tested, and possibly variations in medical training, experience and expectations. Body weight averaged 81.6 kg in the clinical men versus 80.2 kg in the industrial men; relative weights were 101.5 per cent and 100 per cent, respectively (Table 5). Although several variables observed during exercise testing showed statistically significant differences because of the large sample sizes, these differences were too small to be of clinical importance.

Because of the small number of coronary events reported in over 3 years of follow-up, the data in these two cohorts were combined for the purposes of this analysis of preliminary experience.

METHODS

Clinical examination and classification of the subjects were performed prior to exercise testing (Table 6). Measurements of cholesterol were available on 772 men, or 28 per cent. (Since there was no difference in the subsequent incidence of coronary events in relation to presence or absence of a cholesterol determination, there was, in retrospect, no apparent biased selection of men for lipid analysis).

Exercise testing was performed voluntarily, with informed consent and professional supervision and monitoring. The multistage treadmill test of maximal exercise used a standard protocol (Table 7) where nearly linear weight-adjusted oxygen requirements for the first 12 minutes had been previously determined. The endpoint of testing was symptom-limited capacity rather than any arbitrary percentage of age-adjusted maximal heart rates. Less than 2 per cent of the tests were stopped because of equipment failures or adverse signs (see Table 6). A single precordial ECG lead, from V_5 position to inferior tip of right scapula, was used to record heart rate, monitor changes in rhythm, ventricular conduction and repolarization. The pattern of ST response, and the duration of sequential changes in recovery were recorded; the definition of an "ischemic" ST depression was one millimeter or more of horizontal or downsloping of segmental depression for at least 0.06 sec in several consecutive beats (Table 8). In the majority of tests, interpretations were reviewed by cardiologists at the registry, and dataphone transmissions of the analog ECG signals were processed by computer averaging and analysis of QRS voltages and five analyses of ST responses. Blood pressure responses were monitored with a clinical sphygomanometer and stethoscope. Symptoms, signs, circulatory and ECG responses, including coding of arrhythmias were recorded on printed forms and then submitted to the computer registry[*]. The functional aerobic impairment, or per cent deviation from average maximal oxygen uptake, adjusted for age, was derived from exercise duration by nomogram (14). Heart rate impairment, or per cent deviation from normal chronotropic capacity, adjusted for age, was derived by regression (16).

[*] Initial cross-sectional differences in functional responses in relation to cardiovascular disease (15) and the separation of probable effects of disease from those of age have been published elsewhere (16).

Although not part of the original methods, peripheral terminals, linked by dial-up telephone to a central computer, were developed to enhance quality control of input data, and to provide immediate functional evaluations and prognostic statements as well as a summary of the data for the participating physicians.

On the basis of date of testing, follow-up mail questionnaires were sent to all subjects annually. They reported whether any morbidity, defined by admission to hospital, or mortality had occurred. With additional information from physicians, medical records, and families, the causes of these events were classified. Three
cardiologists reviewed all mortality data and classified deaths as sudden cardiac
(within 1 hour or from 1 to 14 hours), non-sudden cardiac deaths, and non-cardiac
deaths. The elapsed time from examination and testing to date of last follow-up
questionnaire, or to death, was calculated for each subject to determine annual
event rates per 1000 men at risk.

Differences in continuous variables were assessed by T-tests, and significance of
differences in event rates, adjusted for elapsed time in months for all subjects,
were considered significant when simultaneous 95 per cent confidence intervals for
the rates were disjoint.

RESULTS

Within approximately three years of follow-up after maximal exercise testing, 38
men (1.4%) developed clinical manifestations of coronary heart disease (Table 9).
Ten in the clinical cohort of men were due to angina pectoris; twenty-three events
were due to myocardial infarction; and 5 were cardiac deaths. Four of the latter
were sudden deaths within one hour. The age-specific incidence of coronary heart
disease events in these men increased progressively with advancing age (Figure 1).

Men who developed coronary events were four years older (Table 10) and they had
slightly higher systolic pressures and heart rates at rest, and elevated cholesterol
concentrations. At submaximal exercise they showed higher systolic and diastolic
pressures and slightly faster heart rates. Pressures were higher at maximal exertion but the more impressive change (P < 0.001) was a reduction in maximal heart
rate. There was a moderate (1-1/2 minutes or 13 per cent) reduction in total exercise duration (P < 0.001). Accordingly, estimated maximal oxygen uptake averaged
30.5 instead of 35.2 ml/kg of body weight/minute. Correcting for a difference in
age, functional aerobic impairment averaged 8.9 per cent, whereas the value in non-
event men was 1.5 per cent. The mean voltage, at one minute after exercise by
computer analysis of ST depression was -0.055 mV in the men who developed events, in
contrast to +0.015 mV in all the others (P < 0.001). Three or more abnormal responses (out of more than 20 listed on worksheet) and 5 per cent or more impairment of
age-adjusted heart rate response to maximal exercise occurred more frequently in the
men who developed coronary events.

The event rates of several possible univariate predictors of subsequent coronary
disease are shown in Figure 2. Of the resting variables, neither age nor occasional
minor ECG abnormalities were significant. The presence of one or more of the conventional risk factors, i.e. positive family history for coronary heart disease,
hypercholesterolemia, hypertension or cigarette smoking, was significantly associated with subsequent coronary events. The failure of hypercholesterolemia by itself
to be significant may be partly attributed to the limited number of measurements.
Hypertension, as classified by the examining physicians, was not significant, yet a
resting systolic pressure of 140 mm Hg or more was a significant predictor. The
history of atypical chest pain, specifically not angina pectoris, was not predictive
of subsequent coronary events.

In contrast, six out of seven univariate exercise variables were significant predictors (Figure 3). Although chest pain was experienced in hardly one per cent of
these men, this was associated with an annual coronary event rate of 55/1000 men.
Next in importance was duration of exercise of less than six minutes, or inability
to complete two stages of this exercise testing protocol.

The sensitivity and specificity of several variables of predictive value arranged in decreasing order of importance (are shown in Table 11). This suggests a slight weighting in favour of one or more of the risk factors. Of the exercise variables, the occurrence of post-exertional ST depression emerges as an important single variable.

Stepwise multivariate analysis of 37 variables identified six with significant association with subsequent coronary heart disease events (Table 12). Only 3 per cent (multiple R^2 = 0.034) of the variation in these events was accounted for by these six variables.

The possibility of using these variables for sequential risk assessment was investigated. In one approach, we looked at the effect of using the risk factors in conjunction with ST response to maximal exercise (Figure 4). In two-thirds of these men who were free of risk factors, an increase in annual coronary heart disease event-rates on the basis of ST depression after maximal exercise was minimal and insignificant. Conversely, for the remaining one-third of the men with one or more risk factors, the events rate was not significantly increased in the absence of ST depression. The combination of one or more risk factors and ST depression, which was observed in 3.5 per cent of this population sample, was associated with a significantly higher ($P < 0.05$) event rate of 27.8/10000 men at risk per year. Whilst the a priori event rate for the over-all sample was 3.9/1000 men, this two-stage assessment differentiated the risks over a range of 2.2 to 27.8/1000 men.

In another approach, we looked at the effect of duration of symptom limited exercise in the presence of chest pain with maximal exercise. As shown in Figure 5, these variables separated men into three groups: (a) 98.2% of the men with duration greater than two stages or 6 minutes and no chest pain had the lowest event rate of 3.2/1000 per year; (b) 1.7% with only one of these two characteristics experienced a significantly higher event rate of 40.4/1000 per year; and (c) 0.1% of the men had shortened duration and experienced chest pain, and the subsequent coronary heart disease event rate was a significantly higher 79.5/1000 per year.

DISCUSSION

There are several unique aspects of this study. First, it is a prospective community study of medical practice. Second, it shows the advantages of exercise testing to the symptomatic limits of functional capacity to enhance the detection of individuals at risk. Third, subjective clinical interpretations of ST responses were usually independently evaluated by computer averaging and analysis. Fourth, periodic follow-up surveillance by mail questionnaires directly to subjects has revealed the subsequent occurrence of coronary heart disease events through 1976.

The 2389 asymptomatic healthy men initially without heart disease, had 27 events within three years, which were due to coronary heart disease (1.1%). Of 372 men with hypertension or atypical chest pain syndromes and without clinical manifestations of heart disease initially, 11 had subsequent events (2.9%, $P < 0.05$). With so few coronary events to date, it is necessary to combine these groups for this preliminary analysis. Accordingly, the annual rate for all these coronary events was 3.9/1000 men at risk. If only myocardial infarction or cardiac deaths were counted, the annual rate was 2.9/1000 men at risk. This rate is 72 per cent of that reported for 214 events in men of 40-58 years of age and 53,800 man-years of observation by the Air Line Pilots Association loss of license insurance program (7).

The fact that 98.2 per cent of 2760 men have had no coronary events in three years indicates a very high proportion of low risk individuals in the Seattle study. Whereas an advisory board recommended expansion of the numbers tested by several thousand persons to provide a larger database, the federal agency supporting the study

promptly reduced the funding to provide for follow-up aspects only. This reflects
the difficulties in mounting a prospective study with scientifically adequate numbers of healthy persons, and the need to examine critically the available evidence
from a study limited by constraints on the sampling requirements.

On the basis of this study design and available data, coronary heart disease events
are more likely to occur in men who have one or more risk factors. Exclusion of
any with manifestations of coronary heart disease on initial clinical examination
reduces the risk of future coronary events to a minimum. If exercise testing is
conducted to symptom-limited capacity, there is an increased risk of subsequent
events due to coronary heart disease in those who experience chest discomfort or
pain, who develop ischemic ST depression, who fail to complete two stages or 6 minutes of this multi-stage protocol, who exhibit three or more abnormal symptoms or
signs or who manifest 5 per cent or more impairment in age-adjusted maximal heart
rate. Inasmuch as heart rate is one of three components of oxygen uptake, this reduction in rate response is at least associated with the observed reduction in exercise duration which is highly correlated with oxygen uptake $(R = +0.9)$ (15). The
increased risk differentiated in nearly two per cent of the healthy men on the basis
of the inability to complete two stages or 6 minutes of this multistage protocol was
unexpected. The oxygen requirement for this level of exertion averages 23 ml/(kg x
min) or about 6.5 times the resting requirement; it is also equivalent to the usual
oxygen requirement for three minutes of exertion with the double Master two-step
test (18). It is important to emphasize that neither this symptom-limited duration
of less than six minutes nor maximal heart rate of less than 95 per cent of age-adjusted normal values can be elicited with any type of submaximal or near-maximal
exercise testing protocol to arbitrary target heart rate limits.

An interesting prospect suggested by these results is the potential value of modified uses of maximal exercise tests in mass screening for early detection of coronary heart disease. Two alternative protocols are proposed (Table 13). Both assume
an initial clinical examination to exclude men with clinical manifestations of coronary disease. In protocol "A", men would also be screened for the presence of
conventional risk factors. In about two-thirds who do not have any risk factors,
and have a low risk of coronary heart disease events within three years, exercise
testing is not likely to be beneficial. In one-third of men with one or more risk
factors, individually supervised maximal exercise testing could identify the 3.5 per
cent with ST depression who have a significantly increased risk for subsequent cardiac events. Concomitantly a large fraction with risk factors do not as yet have a
substantial risk for subsequent coronary events. Sensitivity with this protocol is
39 per cent, specificity 88.5 per cent and predictive risk ratio 4.6 : 1. In the
alternative protocol "B", men without clinical manifestations of heart disease could
be referred for group-supervised multistage exercise testing. If testing were equivalent to completing at least two stages of this multistage protocol and without the
occurrence of chest pain at higher workloads, it would indicate a low risk for developing heart disease within three years. The few who were unable to complete the
test, which represents maximally tolerated exertion for them, and/or who developed
chest pain should be individually tested by a physician for further evaluation of
ECG and blood pressure responses. Although administration of such mass exercise
tests would require the presence of a medical team at the testing site, the costs
of conducting such tests are likely to be relatively small. This protocol has a
sensitivity of 21 per cent, a specificity of 98.5 per cent and a predictive risk
ratio of 14.4 : 1. Although most of the coronary events occur among the false negative responders, the testing procedure does identify a small fraction who were not
detected by the prior clinical examination and who actually have a much higher probability of developing clinical events within three years. Subsequent retesting of
those without these two responsive criteria could identify some who have had progression of latent coronary vascular or myocardial disease with conversion to one or
more positive responses to symptom-limited maximal exercise.

CONCLUSIONS

When clinical examination of middle-aged men fails to detect manifestations of
coronary heart disease, exercise testing to symptom-limited capacity identifies
those who already are at increased risk for such disease. In addition to ST depression, other predictors include reduction of exercise duration, unexpected occurrence of chest pain, reduced chronotropic capacity and occurrence of three or more
abnormal responses. In the absence of conventional risk factors, such testing probably is not necessary. With one or more risk factors, ischemic ST depression
identifies less than 4 per cent with 7-times greater risk of coronary events within
3 years. Duration of such exercise of less than 6 minutes, or chest pain with testing identifies less than 2 per cent with 12 times greater risk for such events.
Conceivably these alternative protocols might offer less costly and more effective
approaches to mass screening for earlier recognition of men at significantly greater risk for myocardial infarction, angina pectoris, or sudden cardiac death, but
the validity of these alternatives to mass screening awaits future demonstration.

REFERENCES

(1) Mattingly, T.W. (1962): Am. J. Cardiol., 9, 395.
(2) Rumball, A. and Acheson, E.D. (1963): Br. Med. J., i, 423.
(3) Robb, G.P. and Marks, H.H. (1967): J.A.M.A., 200, 918.
(4) Doyle, J.T. and Kinch, S.H. (1970): Circulation, 41, 545.
(5) Blackburn, H.W., Taylor, H.L. and Keys, A. (1970): Am. J. Cardiol., 25, 85
     (Abstract).
(6) Blackburn, H.W., Taylor, H.L. and Keys, A. (1970): Circulation, 41, Suppl. 1,
     154.
(7) Doan, A.E., Peterson, D.R., Blackmon, J.R. and Bruce, R.A. (1965): Am. Heart
     J., 69, 11.
(8) Li, Y.-B., Ting, N., Chiang, B.-N., Alexander, E.R., Bruce, T.A. and Grayston,
     J.T. (1967): Am. J. Cardiol., 20, 541.
(9) Bruce, R.A. and McDonough, J.R. (1969): Bull. N.Y. Acad. Sci., 45, 1288.
(10) Aronow, W.S. and Cassidy, J. (1975): Circulation, 52, 616.
(11) Report of a Technical Group on Exercise Electrocardiography (1968): Am. J.
     Cardiol., 21, 871.
(12) Froelicher, V.F., Jr., Yanowitz, F.G. and Thompson, A.J. (1973): Circulation,
     48, 597.
(13) Bruce, R.A. (1974): Circulation, 50, 1.
(14) Bruce, R.A., Kusumi, F. and Hosmer, D. (1973): Am. Heart J., 85, 546.
(15) Bruce, R.A., Gey, G.O., Cooper, M.N., Fisher, L.D. and Peterson, D.R. (1974):
     Am. J. Cardiol., 33, 459.
(16) Bruce, R.A., Fisher, L.D., Cooper, M.N. and Gey, G.O. (1974): Am. J. Cardiol.,
     34, 757.
(17) Kulak, L.L., Wick, R.L., Jr. and Billings, C.E. (1971): Aerospace Med., 6,
     670.
(18) Blackburn, H., Winkler, C. and Vilandre, J. et al. (1970). In Medicine and
     Sport, Vol. 4, Physical Activity and Aging. Eds. Bruner, D. and Jokl, E.
     Basel, Karger, p. 28.

TABLE 1

```
JUSTIFICATIONS FOR/LIMITATIONS OF EXERCISE TESTING


1.  ST DEPRESSION AFTER SUBMAXIMAL EXERCISE STRESS (DOUBLE
    MASTER TWO-STEP, TREADMILL, STAIR-CLIMBING) IDENTIFIES
    SOME INDIVIDUALS AT RISK FOR FUTURE CORONARY HEART
    DISEASE EVENTS.
    (MATTINGLY, 1962, ROBB AND MARKS, 1967, RUMBALL AND
    ACHESON, 1963, DOYLE AND KINCH, 1970; IN U.S. MEN,
    NOT IN NON-U.S. COHORTS (BLACKBURN ET AL., 1970).

2.  MAXIMAL TREADMILL VERSUS STEP TEST INCREASES
    PREVALENCE OF ST DEPRESSION (DOAN ET AL., 1965),
    EVEN IN LOW-RISK CHINESE MEN (LI ET AL., 1967);
    SENSITIVITY FOR DETECTION OF SUBSEQUENT CORONARY
    EVENTS (BRUCE AND McDONOUGH, 1969, ARONOW ET AL., 1971);
    BUT THERE IS EXCESSIVE OBSERVER VARIABILITY (BLACKBURN,
    1968); AND PROPORTION OF FALSE POSITIVES EXCEEDS TRUE
    POSITIVES BY ARTERIOGRAPHIC CRITERIA (FROELICHER, 1973).
```

TABLE 2

```
                POSTEXERTIONAL ST DEPRESSION


1.  NON-SPECIFIC IMBALANCE BETWEEN

    -- CORONARY SUPPLY OF OXYGENATED BLOOD (HEMATOCRIT,
       O₂ SATURATION AND DETERMINANTS OF FLOW)
       AND HEMODYNAMIC STRESS OF SUBENDOCARDIUM (PRIMARILY
       HEART RATE AND SYSTOLIC PRESSURE)

2.  AMOUNT/FREQUENCY ALSO VARIES WITH

    -- SEX, AGE, HYPERTROPHY, CONDUCTION DISORDERS

    -- CORONARY/MYOCARDIAL DISEASE

    -- HYPOKALEMIA, DIGITALIS, OTHER DRUGS

3.  RELIABILITY LIMITED BY

    -- SUBJECT AND OBSERVER VARIABILITY, BUT ENHANCED
       BY COMPUTER AVERAGING/ANALYSIS

4.  SENSITIVITY/SPECIFICITY

    -- FOR DIAGNOSIS AND PROGNOSIS
       VARY WITH SAMPLING, STRESS METHODS AND CRITERIA
```

TABLE 3

```
┌─────────────────────────────────────────────────────────────────┐
│                        STUDY DESIGN                               │
│                                                                   │
│   1.   SELECTED SAMPLING FROM BOTH INDUSTRIAL AND                 │
│        CLINICAL POPULATIONS.                                      │
│                                                                   │
│   2.   PRELIMINARY CLINICAL EXAMINATION AND CLASSIFICATION.       │
│                                                                   │
│   3.   MONITORED RESPONSES TO PROGRESSIVE EXERCISE STRESS         │
│        TO FUNCTIONAL LIMITS.                                      │
│                                                                   │
│   4.   ANNUAL FOLLOW-UP SURVEILLANCE FOR SUBSEQUENT               │
│        MANIFESTATIONS OF CORONARY HEART DISEASE EVENTS.           │
│                                                                   │
└─────────────────────────────────────────────────────────────────┘
```

TABLE 4

SELECTION OF 2760 MEN FOR STUDY		
COHORTS	INDUSTRIAL	CLINICAL
PERSONS EXAMINED/TESTED	2064	5833
MEN, WOMEN EXCLUDED[*]	-316	-4821
MEN SELECTED WITH FOLLOW-UP SURVEILLANCE		
HEALTHY	1632	757
HYPERTENSIVE[**]	93	123
ATYPICAL PAIN SYNDROMES[**]	23	132
SUBTOTALS (ROW PERCENTAGES)	1748 (63.3%)	1012 (36.7%)
COLUMN PERCENTAGES	84.7%	17.3%

[*] WOMEN, MEN WITH CORONARY HEART DISEASE, PRIOR SURGERY, OR NO FOLLOW-UP

[**] WITHOUT POSSIBLE, PROBABLE OR DEFINITE HEART DISEASE

TABLE 5

INITIAL FINDINGS IN TWO COHORTS OF NON-CORONARY HEART DISEASE MEN			
	INDUSTRIAL	CLINICAL	P
NUMBERS	1748	1012	
AGE, YEARS	44.5 ± 7.4	45.2 ± 9.0	< 0.05
HEIGHT, CM	178.6 ± 6.4	178.6 ± 6.6	
WEIGHT, KG	80.3 ± 9.0	81.6 ± 11.3	< 0.001
RELATIVE WEIGHT, %	100.0 ± 9.6	101.5 ± 12.3	< 0.001
CHOLESTEROL, MG/DL	230 ± 42 (N=332)	238 ± 46	< 0.05
SYSTOLIC PRESSURE, MM HG	125 ± 13	124 ± 16	< 0.05
DIASTOLIC PRESSURE, MM HG	79 ± 10	80 ± 10	
HEART RATE	73 ± 11	74 ± 12	< 0.001
ST_B, MV	$+ .05 \pm .06$	$+ .05 \pm .08$	
SUBMAXIMAL EXERCISE (STAGE I, 3rd MINUTE)			
SYSTOLIC PRESSURE, MM HG	156 ± 20	152 ± 22	NS
DIASTOLIC PRESSURE, MM HG	78 ± 11	81 ± 10	NS
HEART RATE	109 ± 14	111 ± 14	NS
MAXIMAL EXERCISE			
SYSTOLIC PRESSURE, MM HG	190 ± 22	184 ± 24	< 0.001
DIASTOLIC PRESSURE, MM HG	71 ± 17	79 ± 16	< 0.001
HEART RATE, B/MIN	182 ± 12	176 ± 16	< 0.001
SP x HR x 10^{-2}	344 ± 43	324 ± 52	< 0.001
DURATION, SEC.	633 ± 90	613 ± 134	< 0.001
EST. OXYGEN UPTAKE ML/(KG x MIN)	35.5 ± 5.0	34.4 ± 7.5	< 0.001
FUNCTIONAL AEROBIC IMPAIRMENT	1.1 ± 11	2.6 ± 16	< 0.01
CHANGE IN HEART RATE, B/MIN	109 ± 14	102 ± 18	< 0.001
HEART RATE IMPAIRMENT, %	0 ± 6	2 ± 7	< 0.001

TABLE 6

METHODS

CLINICAL EXAMINATION/CLASSIFICATION

-- HISTORY, PHYSICAL, ECG, CHEST X-RAY

-- RISK FACTORS (LIPIDS NOT REQUIRED)

MULTISTAGE TREADMILL TEST (BRUCE PROTOCOL)

    (VOLUNTARILY, WITH INFORMED CONSENT)

-- TO FATIGUE OR SYMPTOMS (NOT TARGET RATES)

-- INTERRUPTED ($<$ 2%) BY EQUIPMENT FAILURES

    OR ADVERSE SIGNS

    -- 3 CONSECUTIVE VENTRICULAR PREMATURE BEATS

    -- ONSET OF ATAXIA GAIT

    -- FALL IN SYSTOLIC PRESSURE BELOW USUAL RESTING LEVEL

MONITORING/RECORDING

-- SYMPTOMS, SIGNS

-- PRECORDIAL ECG (CB_5)

    RATE, RHYTHM, CONDUCTION CHANGES

    ST RESPONSES

    (DATAPHONE TRANSMISSION/COMPUTER AVERAGING-ANALYSIS)

-- BLOOD PRESSURE RESPONSES

-- TALLY OF NORMAL, QUESTIONABLE, ABNORMAL ITEMS

-- SCORING OF FUNCTIONAL IMPAIRMENT (AEROBIC, LV, HR)

COMPUTER REGISTRY FILE

-- CROSS-SECTIONAL DIFFERENCES

-- LONGITUNDINAL CHANGES

-- PERIODIC MORBIDITY/MORTALITY SURVEILLANCE

    BY MAIL QUESTIONNAIRES TO SUBJECTS

    AND SUPPLEMENTARY INFORMATION

    FOR CLASSIFICATION OF EVENTS/ANALYSIS

TABLE 7

	"SEATTLE HEART WATCH" TREADMILL TESTING PROTOCOL				
STAGE	SPEED (MPH)	GRADIENT (%)	MINUTES*	APPROXIMATE O_2 COST**	
REST	0	0	0	4	
I	1.7	10	3	17	
II	2.5	12	6	25	
III	3.4	14	9	34	
IV	4.2	16	12	44	
V	5.0	18	15	56	

* EACH STAGE IS 3 MINUTES LONG

** O_2 COST IN ML OF OXYGEN/KG/MINUTE (MEN)

TABLE 8

CLASSIFICATION OF ST RESPONSES TO MAXIMAL EXERCISE

(BASED UPON CLINICAL OR VISUAL INTERPRETATION)

I. NO SIGNIFICANT ST DEPRESSION

II. ST DEPRESSION OF ONE MILLIMETER OR MORE FOR AT LEAST .06 SEC AND FOR SEVERAL CONSECUTIVE BEATS

    1. BORDERLINE - WITH UPSLOPING SEGMENTAL DEPRESSION

    2. ISCHEMIC - WITH HORIZONTAL OR DOWNSLOPING SEGMENTAL DEPRESSION

        A. TRANSIENTLY FOR 1-2 MINUTES

        B. PERSISTENT, AND EVOLVING FOR 3 OR MORE MINUTES AFTER EXERTION

    3. ACCENTUATED DIGITALIS EFFECT

III. ST ELEVATION OF ONE-HALF MILLIMETER OR MORE

TABLE 9

SUBSEQUENT CHD EVENTS REPORTED BY SURVEILLANCE			
COHORTS	INDUSTRIAL	CLINICAL	
NONE	1729 (99.1%)	980 (97.8%)	2709 (98.2%)
MORBIDITY (HOSPITAL ADMISSION)	0.7%	2.1%	1.19%
ANGINA PECTORIS	0	10	10
BY-PASS SURGERY FOR ANGINA	0	0	0
MYOCARDIAL INFARCTION	9	11	20
RECURRENT INFARCTION	3	0	3
SUDDEN CARDIAC ARREST	0	0	0
MORTALITY	0.17%	0.19%	0.18%
SUDDEN CARDIAC	3	1	4
NON-SUDDEN CARDIAC	0	1	1
NON-CARDIAC (EXCLUDED)	4	9	13
CHD EVENTS	15	23	38
CASE FATALITY, %	20.0	9.1	13.9

TABLE 10

DIFFERENCE IN CONTINUOUS VARIABLES			
	NON-EVENT MEN	CORONARY EVENT MEN	P
NUMBER	2722	38	
AGE, YEARS	44.6 ± 7.9	49.1 ± 7.9	< 0.001
WEIGHT, KG	80.8 ± 9.9	78.6 ± 9.0	NS
RELATIVE WEIGHT, %	101 ± 11	99 ± 9	NS
CHOLESTEROL, MG/DL	234 ± 44 (N=754)	262 ± 45 (N=15)	< 0.05
SYSTOLIC PRESSURE, MM HG	124 ± 14	132 ± 19	< 0.01
DIASTOLIC PRESSURE, MM HG	79 ± 10	83 ± 11	< 0.05
HEART RATE, B/MIN	73 ± 12	79 ± 13	< 0.01
ST_B, MV	.05 ± .06	.02 ± .04	< 0.05
SUBMAXIMAL EXERCISE (STAGE I, 3rd MINUTE)			
SYSTOLIC PRESSURE, MM HG	154 ± 21	168 ± 26	< 0.001
DIASTOLIC PRESSURE, MM HG	79 ± 11	85 ± 12	< 0.001
HEART RATE, B/MIN	109 ± 14	114 ± 12	< 0.05
MAXIMAL EXERCISE			
SYSTOLIC PRESSURE, MM HG	188 ± 23	194 ± 32	NS
DIASTOLIC PRESSURE, MM HG	74 ± 17	85 ± 14	< 0.001
HEART RATE, B/MIN	180 ± 13	170 ± 17	< 0.001
HR x SP x 10^{-2}	337 ± 47	331 ± 70	NS
DURATION, SEC.	627 ± 108	543 ± 138	< 0.001
EST. $\dot{V}_{O_2 MAX}$, ML/(KG x MIN)	35.2 ± 6.1	30.5 ± 7.7	< 0.001
FUNCTIONAL AEROBIC IMPAIRMENT, %	1.5 ± 13	8.9 ± 20	< 0.001
HEART RATE IMPAIRMENT, %	0.5 ± 6.0	4.0 ± 8.8	< 0.01
ST_B AFTER EXERCISE, MV			
IMMEDIATELY	-0.031 ± 0.087	-0.079 ± 0.100	< 0.001
1 MINUTE	0.012 ± 0.076	-0.040 ± 0.093	< 0.001
5 MINUTES	-0.019 ± 0.062	-0.046 ± 0.055	< 0.01

TABLE 11

COMPARATIVE VALUE OF CHD PREDICTORS			
	SENSITIVITY %	SPECIFICITY %	INDEX OF MERIT*
ANY ONE OR MORE CONVENTIONAL RISK FACTORS	60.5	67.0	.27
CIGARETTE SMOKING	44.7	81.4	.26
ST DEPRESSION AFTER MAXIMAL EXERCISE	31.6	92.7	.25
HEART RATE IMPAIRMENT ⩾ 5% (MAXIMAL HEART RATE < 95% OF AGE-ADJUSTED AVERAGE NORMAL)	44.7	80.4	.25
FUNCTIONAL AEROBIC IMPAIRMENT ⩾ 20%	26.3	93.3	.19
DURATION OF MAXIMAL EXERCISE < 6 MIN	10.5	99.1	.10
ANY ONE OR MORE RISK FACTORS AND ST DEPRESSION ⩾ 3 MIN	39.1	90.1	.29

*INDEX OF MERIT = $\dfrac{(\text{PER CENT SENSITIVITY} + \text{PER CENT SPECIFICITY}) - 100}{100}$

TABLE 12

VARIABLES IDENTIFIED BY STEPWISE MULTIVARIATE DISCRIMINANT ANALYSIS		
VARIABLES SELECTED	F VALUE	MULTIPLE R^2
1. DURATION OF EXERCISE	22.7	0.0121
2. EXERTIONAL CHEST PAIN	13.5	0.0192
3. AGE	9.0	0.0240
4. FUNCTIONAL AEROBIC IMPAIRMENT	6.8	0.0275
5. RELATIVE WEIGHT	6.0	0.0307
6. HYPERTENSION	6.5	0.0341

TABLE 13

APPROACHES TO MASS SCREENING OF CORONARY HEART DISEASE RISK IN
MEN OF 30 - 64 YEARS OF AGE

STAGE I   - PRIOR CLINICAL EXAMINATION TO EXCLUDE ANY WITH MANIFESTATIONS OF
            HEART DISEASE

STAGE II - ALTERNATIVE PROTOCOLS:

A.

1. EXCLUDE 66% WITHOUT CONVEN-
    TIONAL RISK FACTORS.

2. INDIVIDUALLY SUPERVISED
    TESTING OF MULTISTAGE
    MAXIMAL EXERCISE OF 34%.

3. ST DEPRESSION IDENTIFIES
    3.5% WITH 7 TIMES GREATER
    RISK.

B.

1. GROUP-SUPERVISED, SUBMAXIMAL
    EXERCISE TESTING, WITHOUT ECG
    MONITORING, FOR AT LEAST TWO
    STAGES OR 6 MINUTES AT WORK-
    LOADS UP TO 6.5 METS, WITH
    IMMEDIATE AVAILABILITY OF A
    PHYSICIAN AND ECG WHEN NEEDED.

2. CHEST PAIN AND/OR SHORTENED
    DURATION IDENTIFIES 1.8% WITH
    12.5 TIMES GREATER RISK.

WHICH IS MORE COST-EFFECTIVE?

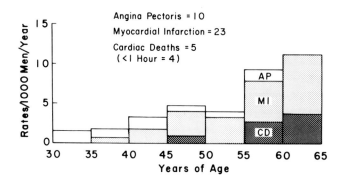

AGE-SPECIFIC INCIDENCE OF
CORONARY HEART DISEASE EVENTS

FIG. 1   Age-specific incidence of coronary heart disease events in men initially
free of clinical manifestations of coronary heart disease. Note increasing
incidence with advancing age.

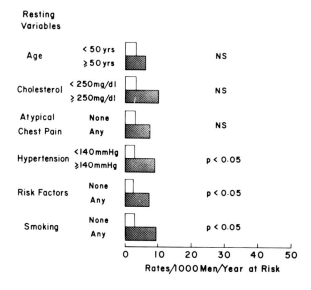

UNIVARIATE PREDICTORS OF CORONARY EVENTS

FIG. 2   Differences in univariate, non-exercise predictors of coronary heart disease events. Note that significance of minor differences in rates depends
upon numbers of men involved as well as event rates.

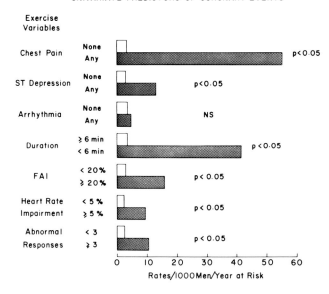

FIG. 3   Differences in univariate exercise predictors of coronary heart disease
          events. Note highest rates in association with chest pain with maximal
          exercise testing, and shortened duration of such testing.

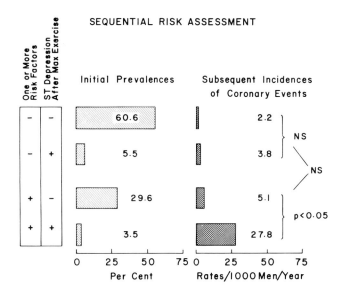

FIG. 4   Interaction of conventional risk factors and ST depression after maximal
          exercise on coronary heart disease event rates. Note that two-thirds of
          the men had no risk factors and that less than four per cent had a
          significantly higher event rate.

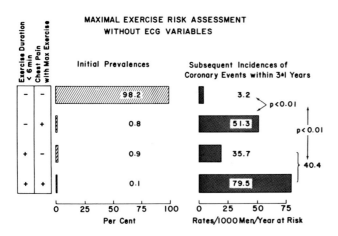

FIG. 5   Interaction of exertional chest pain with maximal exercise testing and
         duration less than 6 minutes on coronary heart disease event rates. Note
         that 98% with neither manifestation had the lowest event rates, whereas
         only 2% had significantly higher rates.

PANEL DISCUSSION ON THE DAY - May 4th

Chairman: Professor John Goodwin

Speakers of the day joined by Dennis Krikler and Clive Layton

(Announcements were made about the Panel Discussions, recording arrangements, etc.)

(1) Professor Goodwin: A question from Dr. J.B. Barlow (Johannesburg). It would
seem to me that the terms "false positive" and "false negative" following
stress testing still require clarification. The ECG changes presumably reflect
myocardial ischaemia, which may or may not be associated with anatomical coronary artery disease. Such cases are therefore not necessarily "false positive"
...
I will not read any more of Dr. Barlow's question or we will get confused.
Perhaps Dr. Coltart would clarify for us the terms "false positive" and "false
negative" ?

Dr. Coltart: Do you want me to say what further techniques one ought to use to
go into it in greater depth? In my presentation I may have missed saying that
with the electrocardiographic analysis of myocardial ischaemia and the ST segment changes, some of the recent studies - in particular, the study from Dr.
Goldschlager and Dr. Selzer's group - have clarified some of the points of
quantitation of the coronary angiogram with ECG changes. When we have a problem with stress test ECG, I believe that if a thallium scan is combined in this
situation the two together may - in general terms - increase the possibility,
or probability of detecting the asymptomatic individual who has latent coronary
artery disease.

Professor Goodwin: Will Dr. Barlow tell us whether Dr. Coltart has answered
his question?

Dr. Barlow: Not entirely. It seems to me that the electrocardiogram reflects
the myocardial ischaemic changes. In the past, prior to thallium studies, the
final arbitrator was often selective coronary arteriography. I find that un-
acceptable because, as we all know, myocardial ischaemia and infarction can
occur with anatomically normal coronary arteries. Conversely, although the
prognosis of abnormal, so-called, ECG changes in women may be very different
from those seen in men, Dr. Bruce has made some observations on the haemodynamic
changes in some women - he found that their pulmonary artery and systemic pressures increased - indicating that although such women presumably have a normal
coronary artery vasculature they may have relative ischaemia, perhaps not of
serious significance but necessarily of a different pattern to that shown in
normal women.

Professor Goodwin: As I see it, the real problem is whether the false positive
or false negative is measuring coronary disease or myocardial ischaemia. Is
that right?

Dr. Barlow: Completely right - and I submit that it is measuring myocardial
ischaemia which may be irrespective of whether or not coronary occlusive disease
is present. Conversely, I submit that there can be a normal stress test but
with significant anatomical coronary artery disease, at which time there is not

significant myocardial ischaemia, possibly because of a good collateral supply.

Dr. Bruce: I agree with Dr. Barlow's interpretation of our report on women. I think it is another piece of evidence for another mechanism contributing to myocardial ischaemia, without necessarily invoking the necessity of coronary vascular disease of that apparent severity. The other part of the problem is that the individuals who we know clinically have symptomatic advanced coronary and myocardial disease with prior infarction, on testing do not show any ST depression, but are negative - apparently falsely negative in this sense. In fact, I am more impressed with other associated observations of poor exercise duration, onset of pain, low heart rate, low blood pressure response - in other words, these patients have much more functional aerobic impairment, left ventricular and heart rate impairment, they have more advanced disease and their prognosis is distinctly worse in our series than others showing rather striking amounts of ST depression.

Again, I emphasise the error of preoccupation with purely ST depression, neglecting everything else. This is contrary to what we try to do in medicine in general, taking into account all the available evidence - history, physical, laboratory data - getting an integrated assessment of it all. We do not identify disease on the basis of a single observation, either very commonly or very reliably.

(2) Professor Goodwin: Question - What apparatus does Dr. Bruce use for his testing? How many episodes of VT/VF have occurred in his total series, and what is the legal position?

I think Dr. Bruce answered those questions in his presentation. Does he want to say anything more?

Dr. Bruce: Serious ventricular arrhythmias, as I mentioned earlier, including ventricular tachycardia, have occurred even in apparently healthy individuals, but with a very low prevalence - about one per cent, or less. So far, these individuals have not had any event. Serious arrhythmia, in the apparent absence of coronary heart disease, is a worrisome, momentary finding, but not necessarily predictive of significant events within three years - it may well in four or five, but nothing has happened within three years to these individuals. The same applies to exertional bundle branch block, for example, that may occur in less than one per cent.

About the legal position, I am not sure that there is any legal hazard when it occurs, whether in the absence or the presence of disease, without any significant event.

On the other hand, when we observe the most lethal type of arrhythmia, namely, ventricular fibrillation, there is now data accrued on about six examples in over 10,000 tests - mostly on coronary patients - and it is interesting to note that these events are post-exertional, within the first one minute or one and a half minutes after stopping exercise. These events occur very early on because they are so symptomatic, always in men who have had a prior clinical diagnosis of coronary heart disease. The recorded data showed that they all had an inadequate rise in systolic blood pressure, or - worse - a fall in blood pressure below the usual resting level during exercise. One of the most important reasons for the physician to be there, to observe, measure or record the blood pressure at frequent intervals is because these are high-risk patients and this is a warning sign that a fatal event can occur. Fortunately, in all these six cases the physician was present and prepared with a defibrillator, all six patients were successfully defibrillated and none has had a myocardial infarction as a result. In this instance, what might have been a disaster six times over has been of no major importance, other than revealing very marked severity of disease. When these individuals were subsequently studied in the arteriographic laboratory, the studies merely confirmed the expected severity of disease, the location and so on, and whether it was feasible to consider other therapy.

Professor Goodwin: We will leave exercise for the moment, but will return to that subject shortly.

(3) Another question - Was there any uptake of Evans blue in the coronary artery system of the pig, or in any other vascular system?

Dr. Schwartz: Yes, the Evans blue dye uptake exhibits a focal distribution in the coronary arteries, in the iliac arteries and so on. We have not studied these specifically, partly because they are much smaller and we wanted to study larger vessels to permit better discrimination of the areas of dye uptake and of no dye uptake.

(4) Professor Goodwin: Dr. K. Bruyneel (Antwerp) asks - Would the members of the panel be so kind as to comment on the way of life and food pattern intake as risk factors, or early precursors to coronary heart disease?

Dr. Slack: It is a difficult question to answer ... (Professor Goodwin agrees) ... My personal view is that alteration in food patterns and way of life, if they are to be directed towards prevention of coronary artery disease, should be specifically chosen to be relevant to the people who are undergoing these changes in their life. People who are not at risk because they have raised cholesterol, or because they cannot tolerate cholesterol in their diet, should not necessarily be singled out because they belong to a nation whose coronary risks are rising to forego cream with strawberries, or butter with their new potatoes. There are many people in the population who can perfectly well indulge in this particular risk factor, whilst smoking may be a particular hazard for them. Preventive measures and the risk factors should be selected which are appropriate to the people who are to undergo them.

Professor Goodwin: With regard to diet, lipids, saturated fats and so on, is there a question of amount? Is it reasonable, for instance, to gorge oneself with saturated fats once a week, provided that the diet is more prudent the rest of the time, or does it not really matter either way?

Dr. Slack: I do not know - I do not have the facts to go on - but probably many people can gorge themselves without having any trouble, whereas there are a few people who are particularly sensitive. These latter are the ones who should avoid them i.e. saturated fats and who probably cannot afford to have too much.

Professor Goodwin: Are we confusing risk factors with markers of disease? We talk rather largely and rather vaguely sometimes about those risk factors. Ought we to distinguish between those things which are in some degree causal and those which are merely incidental and just indicate that disease may be present?

Dr. Slack: I think that there has been a fairly precise definition of risk factors. They are, I believe, those which in a prospective study have proved to identify people who are at increased risk - that is the research I have chosen to talk about ...

Professor Goodwin: You have used the words "risk factor" in the sense of a marker? ... (Dr. Slack agrees) ... Could you tell us which of the many risk factors quoted - not necessarily those you have quoted, but those which are quoted by different people - are really important in terms of being causal to some extent, or of adding risk?

Dr. Slack: I do not know quite what you mean by "causal". There are a limited number of risk factors which fit into the definition of "risk factor" - the definition we have now made. These are:

1. Smoking, which is alone in that there is an improvement in prognosis if it is removed.
2. Cholesterol and blood pressure, both of which have stood up to several tests.
3. Triglycerides, which have only rather marginally been shown in one large study of which I know to be a true risk factor. I am not sure that evidence has been confirmed.

I may be ignorant, but I know of no others.

Professor Goodwin: Smoking is really the independent one?

Professor Mitchell: I wonder whether it would be possible to approach the question of risk factors, or risk markers in another way. Is it not true that there are assumptions and thoughts in people's minds which have not been critically examined? First, leaving aside genetic hyperlipidaemics, in the free-range, normal population diet controls their serum cholesterol level. I know of a lot of studies - Tecumseh, Framingham and so on - which show that although there are differences between Dutchmen, Germans and so on as groups, the individual variation within those groups does not relate to diet. If we were to take all the people in this room, there is no evidence that their serum cholesterol level is set at a particular height by what they eat. Thus, diet as a regulatory factor must be questioned.

The risk factor/risk marker aspect comes back to how we prove these things. Suppose I said that Irishmen eat a lot of potatoes, Irishmen get tuberculosis, therefore tuberculosis results from eating potatoes. A simple way to prove this would be to mount an intervention study to show whether tuberculosis can be prevented by altering potato eating habits. There is no study, currently known to me, which reveals that changing dietary habits will alter life expectancy.

The two questions which must be resolved, apropos of markers versus factors are:

1. The belief that diet controls free-range lipids - free-range cholesterol - has not really stood critical examination.
2. There is no successful intervention study that has been mounted which allows us to move from the marker to the causal factor. There have been three which have attempted to do so:
   (a) The anti-coronary club of New York - a brave try, but not a good statistical exercise.
   (b) Seymour Dayton - he said himself that he had not proved anything.
   (c) The Finnish Mental Hospitals' study - people cannot be put into a mental hospital to do a dietary trial.

Professor Goodwin: It really seems, therefore, that stopping smoking is perhaps the most prudent way of life according to the Panel.

Dr. Kottke: Perhaps I might enlarge slightly on Professor Mitchell's comments. He need not have excluded the hyperlipoproteinaemics because if they are considered as a group there are a couple of other important factors which are commonly overlooked. First, there are marked differences in the way in which people with different lipid disorders handle cholesterol, in terms of excretion rates - from a Type IIa, which handles it poorly and retains cholesterol, to a Type IV, which excretes large amounts of it. Hence, the response to diet of each of these types also varies markedly. One of the problems in previous studies has been that there has not been this separation of individual response on the basis of metabolic disorders, which may perhaps play a more important role than any dietary factors.

Professor Goodwin: Dr. Lawson McDonald has just reminded me that in the United States the number of deaths from coronary disease is falling - I do not know whether this is due to change in diet, or less smoking, or better control of blood pressure, all three or something else. Would anyone on the Panel like to comment on that statement? It is true, is it not, that the incidence in the States is falling? ... (inaudible comment from the Floor) ... I think the figures are right, but I do not know the reason for it ...

Professor Resnekov: It is the incidence of deaths that is falling not necessarily the prevalence of heart disease ...

Professor Goodwin: The incidence of coronary disease is not falling?

Professor Resnekov: We do not know - we think that it might be ...

Professor Goodwin: Perhaps Dr. Selzer would like to comment on it?

Dr. Selzer (San Francisco): I have nothing to add with regard to the risk factors. I agree with Professor Resnekov that it is the deaths that are falling, and I certainly would not give any credit to surgeons in the United States! (Laughter)

(5) Professor Goodwin: The next question is about quantitative angiography and its sensitivity re intravascular thrombus. I am not sure I understand what that means. Can the questioner please amplify it? ... Or perhaps someone on the Panel may understand the questioner better than I?

Professor Blankenhorn: Let me re-phrase the question, then I might be able to answer it. Can one distinguish between an atheroma and an intravascular thrombus? That has not been tested extensively, but we believe such a distinction can be made. Obviously, that test has to be done at a time when the vessel can be angiogrammed and examined so that a predicted/found experiment can be done. The way that we have currently been using the available autopsy material is, first, to wash out the clots to avoid the problem. We have not extensively tested the ability to discriminate between a thrombus on top of a lesion and a lesion itself.

We can begin to discriminate the combination of an ulcerated lesion with clots in it, because of its characteristic shape, from an uncomplicated stenosis. The discrimination of such lesions, I think, will be adequate, but insufficient cases have been done to give an adequate estimate of sensitivity and specificity for that kind of discrimination.

(6) Professor Goodwin: There are some more questions on exercise and stress testing. First, any information on stress other than exercise?

Dr. Coltart: We have had some reports from Taggart and co-workers who monitored people taking sauna baths and undergoing various other activities, such as racing drivers, people driving around London and so on. The study that comes to my mind most readily is that of people driving around London, although I think there was the same trend with middle-aged men having a sauna bath, or people monitored during air flight. Characteristic ECG changes were shown in the subjects, going from normality into what we would recognise as an ischaemic trace during these stresses. Professor Stanley Taylor has also studied stress in this sort of set-up - perhaps he would like to amplify my remarks ...? (Professor Taylor was not then present)

Dr. Bruce: It is true that many different types of stress may initiate this type of response. I recall at one phase we were monitoring patients in the coronary care unit post-infarction. We were struck by the fact that at different times we would unexpectedly see rather striking ST segment changes - T wave changes - in their precordial lead. A nurse kept a log of what happened moment by moment. From this, we learnt that it was totally unpredictable what would stress any given patient. One patient, for example, a member of our faculty, had shown no abnormality four days after infarction, and his wife had visited him frequently. On one particular visit, after she had been there about 20 minutes, she opened her purse, pulled out some papers, said that she did not quite understand the date of those insurance policies and could he please explain? He looked at the papers, answered her factually as though nothing had happened - and he had 3 mm of ST depression for exactly two minutes. He was unaware of any symptoms, had no arrhythmia, nor could he account for it when I confronted him with the evidence later. He did not even associate it with this experience - yet, apparently, this was a stressful experience to him, as seen by the myocardium.

Dr. Layton: I think one or two people were slightly disappointed by the sensitivity and specificity of the exercise testing as a predictor. Of course, coronary disease is a dynamic disorder, not a static situation. It may be that with repetitive testing, say, at yearly intervals, a number of patients who suffer coronary events and who were not predicted at an earlier stage might become predictable. This might perhaps upset cost-effective equations, or protocols at the end. Do you feel that repetitive annual testing is a practical possibility, and would it help?

Dr. Bruce: I, too, have been disappointed by the low sensitivity. As pointed out by Dr. Coltart on one of his slides, as well as in the literature, the prevalence of this response depends on the population sampled. If the population is healthy, asymptomatic individuals, the prevalence will be even lower - we also have found that. In terms of re-testing, from our earlier pilot study data, in one group of over 200 individuals that we followed on repeated annual testing over about eight years, we observed the fact that on each examination the prevalence of ST depression increased. It seemed to be rising progressively. Is this a non-specific effect of age - because they were growing older, year by year? Certainly, there is a strong relationship with age. Alternatively, is it evidence of disease? Curiously, however, it seemed to be related to both and, again, it is hard to sort out - the population sample was not sufficiently large for us to be able to answer this question satisfactorily.

We are in the process now of looking at it, in terms of re-testing. Data are accumulating on over 1,000 individuals and we hope we will obtain a rather more specific answer.

(8) Dr. Layton: A questioner asks - Could you provide some more detailed information on the age composition and age-specific rates of ST depression? Did you find any clinical differences between individuals with and without ST depression, in respect of blood pressure, cholesterol levels and so on? I think some

of that information was given in your presentation.

Dr. Bruce: In looking at this we have found that the prevalence of ST depression - the ischaemic definition - goes up with each five-year subdivision of a age, both in the healthy group and in the patients. The difference between the two groups is roughly the same for all age groups from 30 to 65 years of age. Years ago, in the pilot study, at the third examination we were struck by the fact that 89 per cent of the individuals had exactly the same response three times running, over a period of three years, the other 11 per cent showing changes. When we investigated further, we found that about an equal number had changed from positive to negative and from negative to positive, also that the changes were associated with variations in terms of cholesterol levels and blood pressure responses which were provocative - this seemed to make sense. There may thus be an association.

More recently, another study, not yet published, has been carried out by one of our young people, in which 56 healthy men from the industrial cohort were investigated. The study was very carefully designed and these individuals were tested again one week later, at the same time of day, same day of the week and in as similar circumstances as could possibly be obtained. In essence, it was found that only about 70 per cent of these individuals had exactly the same response - whether positive or negative - one week later. There certainly is a great deal of variation in the same individuals from one time to another, with exactly the same testing and apparently the same circumstances, which is not yet accounted for. Again, this emphasises that there are many different factors which contribute to the response. We think that in many people it is related to coronary disease, but other facts must also be taken into account.

(9) Professor Goodwin: Professor Maseri asks - What is the prognosis and evaluation of the patient with angina at rest and normal exercise capacity?

Dr. Coltart: (doubtful about the question)

Professor Goodwin: Is this a non-sequitur?

Dr. Coltart: Angina at rest and normal exercise capacity - presumably, therefore, he cannot exercise because he has angina at rest: Could Professor Maseri enlarge ...

Professor Goodwin: Perhaps Professor Maseri would clarify the question.

Professor Maseri: I do not know whether this is unique to our patients, but we have many patients who tell us they have angina at rest - and this is quite typical angina. The resting ECG is normal, they are exercised and do well, yet they may have angina when they are shaving - in the afternoon, however, they can play tennis or chop wood. I wonder what can be done for these patients ...

Dr. Coltart: (intervening) ... and you do a thallium scan which is normal. You are "billing" me up to say that it is coronary spasm - which you will discuss tomorrow!

Professor Goodwin: I am rather scared to do exercise testing on people with angina at rest - but obviously it can be done. Have you any comments on it, Professor Mitchell? (No). Professor Holland? (No).

(10) There is a second part to Professor Maseri's question: what is the prognosis and evaluation of the patient with angina and normal or minimal coronary stenosis?

Dr. Bruce: This is in terms of symptomatic angina pectoris and minimal coronary artery stenosis ...

Professor Goodwin: (intervening) ... It is our old friend, angina with normal coronary arteries, is it not - whatever that may be? (Professor Maseri nods agreement)

Dr. Bruce: I am intrigued by the fact that in a coronary patient group - not the group I described earlier this afternoon - when we look at their exercise responses there is a remarkable gradient for future risk of cardiac death on only three variables:

1. Cardiomegaly - which occurs in eight per cent.

2. Duration of less than three minutes, or unable to reach Stage 2 of this protocol of testing.

3. A peak systolic pressure during exercise below 130 mm mercury.

Curiously, about 73 per cent (about 1,600 patients) of these coronary patients have none of these three. These have the lowest risk of all the coronary patients: 20 per 1,000 per year. Thus, three out of four have low risk. I suspect that these are often the patients that physicians and surgeons treat and in whom they obtain, and report, excellent results. They do well anyway.

On the other hand, those patients with any one of the three variables have a mortality risk of 95 per 1,000 per year; for those with any two, the risk is about 250 per 1,000 per year, and the 0.5 per cent that have all three variables are at extreme risk, with a mortality rate of 880 per 1,000 per year. In comparison, the earlier data reported from the Cleveland Clinic on invasive studies, three-vessel disease, low ejection fraction, showed 85 per cent mortality in five years. Here, with non-invasive variables, from exercise testing with this protocol, available on the first examination in the doctor's office, there is this ability to differentiate the very high-risk patient in one year.

Professor Goodwin: The next question demands a fairly quick answer.
(11) Dr. Douglas-Jones (Norfolk) - Is there any evidence that high-density lipoproteins protect against myocardial infarction?

Dr. Slack: I do not think there has been any prospective study on this yet - I am unaware of any such study. From what we know about high-density lipoproteins in people of different races, in women as compared with men, and the changes found in women on the contraceptive pill, it would indicate that this may be a fruitful line of investigation.

Professor Goodwin: Do you agree with that Professor Mitchell? (Apparently he does)

Dr. Schwartz: Relevant to this is the work of Brown and Goldstein which shows - this may be relevant to the pathogenesis of the disease - that high-density lipoprotein can prevent the binding and the internalization of low-density lipoproteins by cells in culture. This is a matter of considerable interest in the biology of atheroma.

Professor Goodwin: Does any other member of the Panel want to comment? ... You all agree ...? (No comments)

(12) Dr. Layton: Dr. Mahon (Massachusetts, U.S.A.) asks - How valid are ST segment changes occurring during exercise in patients who are on digitalis, regardless of the digitalis effect on the resting electrocardiogram?

Dr. Bruce: If one is considering the possibility of making a diagnosis of myocardial ischaemia and coronary disease, this virtually excludes the opportunity unless the individual is re-tested several days after he has the chance to excrete whichever compound has been used to see whether or not the same type of response occurs.

If, however, it is turned round the other way, looking at it in terms of prognosis, our data clearly show in coronary patients who are digitalised and have what we call an accentuated digoxin effect, with even more ST depression during exercise than they showed at rest, that this is an important prognostic indicator of mortality. This should not come as a surprise because the patients who are usually treated with one of these glycosides are usually further along the course of their coronary disease, and have clinical manifestations of arrhythmias that might be appropriate for treatment, or, more commonly, heart failure.

(13) Professor Goodwin: I should like each member of the Panel to give a quick answer to the following question. What kind of a message have you for the general practitioner after this first day?

Dr. Slack: May I suggest that he looks out for the high-risk groups which have been identified today, as far as he can manage.

Professor Blankenhorn: To follow on from Dr. Slack's comments, in examining the vessels serially of high-risk patients with hyperlipoproteinaemia we have found some evidence that the rate of change towards regression is directly proportional to lipid level: the lower the triglyceride and the cholesterol the more likely the lesion is to change in a favourable direction, and conversely, the higher the level the more likely to show progression.

Dr. Coltart: Hopefully, to be aware of the problems with all the methodology and predictive values and markers that are present. If general practitioners are aware of the problems, perhaps they can co-operate with the studies so that we might make some advances to answer these various problems.

Dr. Kottke: My message is not to be too anxious to wait for the epidemiological studies because I think it will be possible in the fairly near future to carry out studies based on arterial wall lesions and their measurements.

Professor Mitchell: Many of the studies that have used complicated methods - including sophisticated methods, such as Dr. Bruce's - have shown that there is still no substitute for taking a good history, a good family history, for doing a proper physical examination which includes measuring and recording the blood pressure, looking at people to see whether they are fat, asking them whether they smoke and, before doing anything else, such as measuring blood lipids or any other sophisticated measurement, telling the patients that they are already neglecting simple precautions which they did not need a doctor to tell them about, but for which they need a doctor to reinforce them about. I think the simple message for all doctors is shown by what came out of the Glasgow screening survey for blood pressure: if only the doctors who had been in contact with the patients during the preceding two to three years had actually taken their blood pressure, whether they were doctors in ophthalmic clinics, gynaecology departments, fracture clinics, general practitioners or whatever, it would have been almost as good as complicated screening.

Although I have taken a little while to say it, my message is straightforward: there is no substitute for ordinary, old-fashioned doctoring - history taking, physical examination and looking at common sense risk factors, the removal of which cannot conceivably do harm. Stopping a smoker smoking, making a fat person thinner - where is the harm in doing that? Screening for lipids, then not knowing what to do with the answers - that is different.

Professor Holland: Professor Mitchell has said most of what I wanted to say. I should like to emphasise that the general practitioners should use the opportunity afforded by the visits made to them by most children, at least once a year. These children are generally taken by somebody. During that confrontation the general practitioner usually deals only with the particular complaint, but he should use that opportunity for other purposes, such as talking to the mother if she is a smoker, talking to her too if the child is overweight. The major message I would give is that the confrontation of doctor/patient is being used at present only for a curative purpose, or a caring purpose, usually ineffectively. Perhaps there ought to be more emphasis on the preventive aspects which at that stage might be more effective than the sort of evangelical approach there is through screening.

Dr. Schwartz: I like an approach which is really a combination of two we have heard about so far. Professor Mitchell's approach is very sound. Personally, I can see little reason why one should not be seriously concerned with the problems of cigarette smoking, of the treatment of hypertension and overweight, with exercise and with moderation in diet in a simple, common sense manner. But what Dr. Slack said, too, is important - to make sure that, as part of the good history that is taken, as suggested admirably by Professor Mitchell, we also have a close look at the family history. There is little doubt that some people have a uniquely high risk, so there is at least some merit in having a close look at such people, making every endeavour to modify whatever the markers present may be, looking at their lipids and lipoprotein levels, and perhaps, making an exceptionally solid effort to do something about them because we know that these people will have a very high mortality rate.

Secondly, to ensure that general practitioners are familiar with the treatment and management of patients with high blood pressure.

Dr. Bruce: I cannot disagree with the previous speakers. Professor Mitchell summed it up beautifully.

I expect the situation is the same here as in the United States, that many physicians are already well aware of the message and are honestly trying to implement it. The problem is not how to reinforce the message to the general practitioners, but that they - and us - need to find out how to motivate people to make changes. I am not sure that we are the right people to do it; we are not trained in these disciplines and will have to turn our attention increasingly for help from the social scientists, psychologists and psychiatrists, whoever it may be who seems to have some understanding of motivation and what makes people stop, listen, pay attention and modify their behavioural patterns, some of which they adopt but many of which they acquire. As Paul White said long ago: "We inherit both the genes and our culture from our parents".

Dr. Layton: At the bottom of this question there may be a feeling which has come through several times today, that having recognised the patient with very early coronary heart disease, apart from advising him to stop smoking, we do not have much hard evidence of an effective remedy at that stage. I suggest that there are few diseases in which effective treatment has preceded an ability to diagnose the condition. As a first step, therefore, it is surely important that we should try to identify these people. Only then can we expect to be able to evaluate which treatment, or which preventive measures will be effective.

Professor Goodwin: May I thank the members of the Panel for their co-operation, the audience for providing us with so many excellent questions and, finally, the Panel again for their tolerance to the amount of speaking they have had to do. (Applause)

RADIOACTIVE TRACERS IN THE EARLY RECOGNITION OF ISCHEMIC HEART DISEASE

Bertram Pitt

Johns Hopkins Medical Institutions, Baltimore, Maryland, U.S.A.

Radioactive tracers are playing an increasing role in the early recognition of ischemic heart disease (1). Three techniques have been found particularly useful and show promise for wide clinical application. (1) Myocardial imaging with thallium-201, (2) infarct avid imaging with technetium 99m pyrophosphate, glucoheptonate, or tetracycline, (3) evaluation of left ventricular function following intravenous injection of technetium 99m human serum albumin by multiple gated acquisition cardiac blood pool imaging (MUGA).

Thallium-201 is the current tracer of choice for detecting myocardial ischemia (2). Thallium-201 is taken up by the normal myocardium in proportion to regional myocardial blood flow in the presence of an active sodium-potassium ATPase transport system (3). Areas of myocardial ischemia or infarction can be detected by the regional absence of tracer uptake "cold spot scan". With this technique areas of myocardial ischemia can be detected within a few minutes after experimental coronary artery occlusion. Studies by Wackers et al. in Amsterdam have suggested that thallium-201 myocardial imaging is a sensitive means of detecting patients with acute myocardial infarction (4). Within the first six hours of onset of infarction almost 100% of nontransmural and transmural infarction can be detected by the finding of a focal area of absent tracer uptake on the thallium-201 myocardial image. After this time the sensitivity for detection of infarct-on diminishes. In our experience approximately 2/3 of patients with nontransmural infarction and approximately 90% of patients with transmural infarction can be detected in the first 24-48 hours following onset of symptoms. Although the sensitivity for detection of infarction by thallium-201 continues to diminish with time it remains signficantly greater than that for the electrocardiogram. In a recent study by Bailey et al. in our laboratory, thallium-201 myocardial imaging detected significantly more patients with a history of myocardial infarction than standard electrocardiographic criteria (5). Although precise quantification of infarct size has not been achieved by current thallium-201 myocardial imaging techniques, the size of the thallium-201 myocardial defect appears to be a useful guide to the extent and location of infarction and therefore to prognosis. A limitation of thallium-201 myocardial imaging has been the inability to distinguish areas of acute ischemia from areas of old infarction. Recent experience with redistribution thallium-201 myocardial imaging has however suggested that this technique may also be useful in distinguishing areas of ischemia from those of old infarction. Studies by Pohost et al. at Massachusetts General Hospital in Boston have shown that following an episode of transient myocardial ischemia the thallium-201 defect detected within the first 30 minutes following onset of ischemia will not be detected if the imaging is repeated 1-3 hours later (6). In a recent study by Pond et al., patients with transient myocardial ischemia, as proven by subsequent serial serum enzymes and electrocardiograms, were found to have an initial thallium 201 myocardial defect which was no longer present 1-3 hours later when imaging was repeated (7). Patients with acute myocardial infarction were found to have an initial thallium-201 myocardial defect, which on reimaging 1-3 hours later either increased in size or diminished slightly but did not disappear. In patients with areas of old myocardial infarction, initial thallium-201 myocardial defects were unchanged 1-3 hours later when imaging was repeated. While experience with this technique is still limited, and exceptions to the above criteria are to be expected, it appears likely that myocardial imaging with thallium-201 will be of value in the early evaluation of patients with suspected acute myocardial infarction.

Perhaps the most exciting use of thallium-201 myocardial imaging is in the evaluation of patients with suspected ischemic heart disease. Studies by Bailey et al. have shown that exercise thallium-201 myocardial imaging is more sensitive than conventional exercise electrocardiography for the detection of myocardial ischemia in patients with angiographically significant coronary artery disease (8). This technique is particularly useful in patients in whom the resting electrocardiogram is abnormal due to an intraventricular conduction defect, left ventricular hypertrophy, digitalis defect, or previous myocardial infarction. The sensitivity for detection of myocardial ischemia increases with the extent of coronary artery narrowing. In patients with significant triple vessel disease approximately 90% of patients can be detected by the combination of rest plus exercise thallium-201 imaging. Although occasional patients with severe triple vessel disease may not be detected by thallium-201 myocardial imaging because the myocardium is diffusely ischemic and hence tracer uptake uniformly reduced, the vast majority of patients with triple vessel disease are easily detectable since one or another vascular area may become ischemic before the other resulting in a focal tracer defect of thallium-201 uptake, the hallmark of myocardial ischemia. Rest plus exercise thallium-201 myocardial perfusion imaging has also proven useful in the localization of the site of myocardial ischemia (5). The greatest sensitivity with current imaging technics is found in patients with left anterior descending or right coronary artery lesions, the least with left circumflex coronary artery lesions. Defects due to the left anterior descending coronary artery are localized in the anterior and apical segments of the anterior thallium-201 image and in the septal region of the 40 and 60° left anterior oblique image. Proximal left anterior descending coronary artery lesions can be separated from distal left anterior descending coronary artery lesions by the finding of a tracer defect in the septal region in the former and only the anterior apical segment in the latter. This differentiation is important since recent angiographic studies by Griffith et al. suggest that patients with significant proximal left anterior descending coronary artery lesions have a worse prognosis and a higher incidence of sudden death than those with distal left anterior descending coronary artery lesions, lesions of the left circumflex, or right coronary artery (9). Right coronary artery lesions can be detected by the finding of a perfusion defect in the inferior segments on the anterior view and the lower lateral segments on the 40° left anterior oblique view. There appears to be considerable overlap of the right coronary artery and left circumflex coronary artery thallium-201 distribution, defects in the high lateral wall in the 60° left anterior oblique thallium-201 image appear however to be fairly specific for narrowing of the left circumflex coronary artery.

Another useful application of thallium-201 myocardial imaging is in the evaluation of asymptomatic patients with a positive exercise electrocardiographic stress test. Over the past few years there has been increasing use of exercise electrocardiography to screen executives, pilots, and asymptomatic patients with one or more cardiac risk factors. A relatively large percentage of positive exercise electrocardiographic stress tests under these circumstances turn out to be falsely positive, in that subsequent arteriography fails to reveal significant anatomic coronary artery disease. The finding of a positive exercise thallium-201 myocardial image in an asymptomatic patient with a positive exercise electrocardiographic stress test increases the likelihood that the patient has significant anatomic coronary artery disease. The finding of a negative exercise thallium-201 myocardial image considerably lessens this possibility, although it does not entirely limit it.

Thallium-201 myocardial imaging is also useful in the evaluation of patients with suspected coronary artery spasm. Injection of thallium-201 during a spontaneous episode of variant angina has been shown to document the presence and site of ischemia by Maseri et al. In patients with suspected coronary artery spasm, thallium-201 myocardial imaging can be performed following IV injection of ergonovine. The finding of an initial thallium-201 myocardial defect that is no longer present 1-3 hours later on the redistribution image is suggestive evidence for the presence of coronary artery spasm. In occasional patients with suspected coronary artery spasm, we have been able to demonstrate episodes of ischemia induced by ergonovine by thallium-201 myocardial imaging but not by standard electrocardiography.

Infarct avid imaging with technetium 99m pyrophosphate is also a sensitive means for detecting patients with acute myocardial infarction (10). In this technique areas of acute infarction are detected by the accumulation of tracer within the area of acute myocardial damage. The mechanism of uptake of tracer by the acutely damaged myocardium is controversial. Although initial studies suggested that uptake of technetium 99m pyrophosphate was due to deposition of calcium within the damaged myocardial cells, more recent studies suggest that the radionuclide may bind non-specificity with the damaged proteins within the myocardial cells. Almost 100% of patients with acute nontransmural and transmural infarction can be detected if imaging is performed 48-72 hours after onset of symptoms (11). Uptake of this radiopharmaceutical in areas of acute infarction appears to be maximal around 48-72 hours and is dependent upon both the time from acute damage and residual myocardial blood flow. Although infarct avid imaging with technetium 99m pyrophosphate has found wide application, its clinical application is limited by the necessity to wait approximately 24-48 hours after the onset of symptoms. By this time the majority of patients with suspected acute myocardial infarction can be diagnosed by serial enzymes and electrocardiographic studies. In the 1/4 to 1/3 of patients seen in the coronary care unit in whom the diagnosis of myocardial infarction is still uncertain at 24-48 hours the availability of an independent technique to detect infarction would be desirable. Unfortunately, it is just in these difficult cases in which this technique is also a problem. For the most part these patients have small nontransmural myocardial infarctions and it may be difficult to be certain of the diagnosis by an technic. There are also an increasing number of false positive diagnoses of myocardial infarction with technetium 99m pyrophosphate. Patients with left ventricular aneurysms, calcific valvular heart disease, cardiomyopathies, and approximately 25% of patients with unstable angina pectoris but without other evidence of myocardial infarction will have a positive technetium 99m pyrophosphate image. Although there appears to be several limitations to the clinical application of this technic, experience with infarct avid imaging with technetium 99m tetracycline and pyrophosphate has provided a valuable basis for future attempts at acute infarct avid imaging in the future. Initial attempts at quantification of infarct size with technetium 99m pyrophosphate have shown a good correlation in both animals and patients with acute anterior transmural infarction but a relatively poor correlation in other situations. Recent tomographic technics do however show promise of allowing the quantification and localization of acute infarction in inferior as well as anterior infarction (12). The group at New York Hospital (13), Cornell Medical Center have recently revived interest in infarct avid imaging with technetium 99m glucoheptonate (14). This radionuclide is also taken up by acutely damaged myocardium but in contrast to technetium 99m pyrophosphate and tetracycline uptake appears to be maximal at approximately 12 hours after onset of infarction. Infarction can be detected by injection of tracer as early as 6 hours after the onset of symptoms. After injection of technetium 99m glucoheptonate imaging should be delayed for approximately 3-5 hours in order to allow adequate clearance of tracer from the blood.

Gated cardiac blood pool imaging after injection of technetium 99m human serum albumin allows estimation of the effect of ischemia and/or infarction on both total and regional left ventricular function (15). Recent modifications of this technic using computer processing allows accumulation of a 28-56 frame isotope angiogram, each frame of which is the sum of several hundred individual beats. These images can be viewed in a cine format similar to standard contrast left ventricular cine angiography. Correlation of left ventricular ejection fraction and regional myocardial wall motion obtained with this technic and standard contrast left ventricular cine-angiography has been excellent. Recent development of semi-automatic edge detection technics allow accurate and reproducible serial noninvasive determination of left ventricular function and regional myocardial wall motion (16). Left ventricular function can be monitored for several hours following a single 10-20 mCi injection of technetium 99m human serum albumin. Studies by Rigo et al. have shown that gated cardiac blood pool imaging is a sensitive means of detecting and localizing areas of myocardial infarction by the detection of areas of regional akinesis. The determination of left ventricular ejection fraction within the first few hours of myocardial infarction by gated cardiac blood pool imaging appears to be a more sensitive means of detecting left ventricular dysfunction than standard hemodynamic measurements including left ventricular filling pressure and cardiac output (17). The effect of therapeutic interventions such as intravenous nitroglycerin in patients with acute myocardial infarction can be easily monitored both acutely and serially. Multiple gated blood pool imaging at rest and during exercise has also been found useful in the detection and evaluation of patients with suspected ischemic heart disease. Borer and his colleagues at the National Institutes of Health in Bethesda, Maryland have shown that normal patients tend to increase their left ventricular ejection fraction during exercise while in those with significant coronary artery disease, left ventricular ejection fraction remains at the same level or decreases during exercise (18). With this technic almost 100% of patients with angiographically proven coronary artery disease could be detected regardless of symptomatology. Although experience with this technique for the detection of ischemic heart disease is still limited, it is clear that the clinician has a new and powerful tool at his disposal for the early detection and evaluation of coronary artery disease.

Used in combination these technics are even more valuable. For example, in patients with cardiogenic shock thallium-201 myocardial imaging reveals a large perfusion defect of the left ventricle and gated cardiac blood pool imaging a large poorly contracting left ventricle in the majority of patients. In occasional patients with electrocardiographic evidence of acute inferior myocardial infarction in cardiogenic shock the thallium-201 myocardial image reveals a relatively small defect in tracer uptake in the left ventricular free wall and the gated cardiac blood pool image a relatively well contracting left ventricle but a large poorly contracting right ventricle. This combination suggests the presence of massive right ventricular infarction (19). Early recognition of this problem and separation of these patients from those with massive left ventricular infarction is important since the prognosis of those with right ventricular infarction is excellent if they are promptly recognized and appropriate therapy instituted. The combination of thallium-201 myocardial imaging and gated cardiac blood pool imaging is also of value in evaluating patients with severe left ventricular failure and/or cardiogenic shock due to papillary muscle rupture or rupture of the interventricular septum. A relatively small infarction as detected by thallium-201 myocardial imaging and/or infarct avid imaging with a good left ventricular ejection fraction suggests a good long term prognosis despite massive failure if the defect can be surgically corrected. An extensive thallium-201 myocardial tracer defect and a low left ventricular ejection fraction suggest a poor prognosis even if surgery is attempted. Thallium-201 myocardial imaging and gated cardiac blood pool imaging are also useful in the pre and postoperative evaluation of patients undergoing coronary artery bypass graft surgery. The appearance of a new resting thallium myocardial tracer defect and a new wall motion abnormality following surgery suggest perioperative infarction (20). Detection of perioperative infarction by the combination of thallium-201 and gated cardiac blood pool imaging or by infarct avid imaging by technetium 99m pyrophosphate has been found to be twice as sensitive as standard electrocardiographic techniques. Postoperative disappearance of a preoperatively detected exercise thallium-201 myocardial defect and improvement in the postoperative left ventricular ejection fraction suggest that the patient's graft is patent and that myocardial perfusion is improved. Studies by Cohen et al. suggest that it may be possible to eliminate postoperative coronary angiography in patients undergoing coronary bypass graft surgery to evaluate graft patency in left ventricular performance in the majority of patients (20).

Clearly we are only at the beginning of a new era in cardiac diagnosis and early recognition of coronary artery disease. With further developments in radiopharmaceuticals, computer processing, and introduction of tomographic gamma tomography, the clinician will soon have at his disposal accurate means of detecting myocardial ischemia, distinguishing ischemia from infarction, quantifying the extent and location of ischemia and/or infarction, the ability to determine the effect of the damaged myocardium on both total and regional left ventricular function, and to assess the effect of therapeutic interventions both acutely and serially.

REFERENCES

(1) Pitt, B. and Strauss, H.W. (1977): Seminars in Nuclear Medicine, 7, 3.
(2) Strauss, H.W. and Pitt, B. (1977): Seminars in Nuclear Medicine, 7, 49.
(3) Strauss, H.W., Harrison, K., Langan, J.K. et al. (1975): Circulation, 51, 641.
(4) Wackers, F.J., Sokole, E.B., Samson, G. et al. (1976): N. Engl. J. Med., 295, 1.
(5) Bailey, I., Burow, R., Griffith, L.S.C. et al. (1977): Am. J. Cardiol., 39, 320.
(6) Pohost, G.M., Zir, L.M., McKusick, K.A. et al. (1977): Circulation, 55, 294.
(7) Pond, M., Rehn, T., Burow, R. et al. (1977): Circulation (In Press).
(8) Bailey, I.K., Griffith, L.S.C., Rouleau, J. et al. (1977): Circulation, 55, 79.
(9) Griffith, L.S.C.: Unpublished observations.
(10) Bonte, F.J., Parkey, R.W., Graham, K.D. et al. (1974): Radiology, 110, 473.
(11) Parkey, R.W., Bonte, F.J., Buja, L.M. et al. (1977): Seminars in Nuclear Medicine, 7, 15.
(12) Keyes, J.: Unpublished observations.
(13) Elfanso: Unpublished observations.
(14) Grossman, M. (1977): Journal of Nuclear Medicine, 18, 548.
(15) Pitt, B. and Strauss, H.W. (1976): Am. J. Cardiol., 38, 739.
(16) Pitt, B. and Strauss, H.W. (1977): N. Engl. J. Med., 296, 1097.
(17) Rigo, P., Strauss, H.W., Taylor, D.R. et al. (1974): Circulation, 50, 678.
(18) Borer, J.: Unpublished observations.
(19) Rigo, P., Murray, M., Taylor, D.R. et al.(1975): Circulation, 52, 268.
(20) Cohen, H., Rouleau, J., Griffith, L. et al. (1975): Circulation, 51 & 52, II, 170.

SUDDEN DEATH

Desmond Julian

University of Newcastle, Newcastle upon Tyne

Sudden unexpected death may occur at almost any time in the course of coronary heart disease. It may complicate both long-standing stable angina pectoris and the acute phase of myocardial infarction but this paper is predominantly concerned with its occurrence in those without known cardiac disease. It has been estimated that sudden death is the first overt feature of coronary heart disease in 15 - 25 per cent of cases (1 - 5).

There is regrettably little information on the precursors of sudden death in those without known heart disease as compared with those with established angina or myocardial infarction. This is unfortunate for it is probable that risk factors are very different.

Pathology of Sudden Death
It is now recognised that most patients dying suddenly of coronary heart disease have at least one, and usually two or three, of the main coronary arteries critically narrowed (3). Transmural infarction appears to be relatively infrequent, although it has been recognised that the patient may die before the pathological appearances of infarction have had time to take place. However, important evidence on this subject is forthcoming from findings in patients who are resuscitated from ventricular fibrillation outside hospital. Cobb and his colleagues (6, 7) from Seattle reported that ECG and enzyme evidence of acute transmural myocardial infarction was observed in only 16 per cent of patients resuscitated from ventricular fibrillation. Coronary angiographic and ventriculographic studies on these patients showed that about one-third have single vessel disease, a further third have two-vessel disease, and the remaining third three-vessel disease. About 50 per cent of patients had reasonable ventricular function in that they had an ejection fraction of more than 50 per cent. It is apparent that a substantial proportion of these patients who were resuscitated had "hearts too good to die" although there was a sub-group, composed largely of those with three-vessel disease and low ejection fractions, who were particularly susceptible to recurrent ventricular fibrillation. Important as these findings are, they only apply to patients who have been resuscitated from ventricular fibrillation. They do not apply to those patients whose cause of death was cardiac rupture, nor to those dying from ventricular fibrillation for whom resuscitation was unsuccessful because of the severity of the underlying myocardial disease. Nonetheless, there can be no doubt that many patients outside Seattle are dying with relatively mild coronary arterial disease and with little myocardial damage. It would clearly be desirable to identify such patients in advance so that prophylactic measures could be undertaken.

The question as to whether thrombosis and myocardial damage are important factors in sudden death remains unanswered. Spain and Bradess (8, 9) and Roberts and Buja (10) have claimed a very low incidence of thrombi (respectively 16 and 8 per cent) in patients dying suddenly. In the study of Adelson and Hoffman (11) 33 per cent of sudden deaths were found to have thrombi with 26 per cent having evidence of acute myocardial infarction. In 63 per cent there were no acute lesions and in 26 per cent the myocardium appeared entirely normal.

Coronary artery spasm is now accepted as a cause of ischaemic heart pain (12), but its importance as a factor in sudden coronary death has not been established.

In recent reports on sudden death, cardiac rupture has been largely ignored. However, it has been stated that myocardial rupture is responsible for approximately 10 per cent of deaths from acute myocardial infarction, being most frequent in the aged and particularly in women (13, 14). Although it may occur on the first day, it commonly occurs later during the first week. It is particularly likely to occur at the junction of old scar and fresh myocardial infarction (14, 15). Although this is a form of sudden death that does not lend itself to resuscitation, it may be to some extent preventable in that hypertension appears to be a factor in its genesis (16).

Mechanism of Sudden Death
Data reported by emergency medical teams which rapidly retrieve patients with "collapse" (17, 18) have proved that a high proportion of patients who are seen soon after the onset of apparent cardiac arrest demonstrate ventricular fibrillation. One cannot be sure that this arrhythmia has not been preceded by a period of asystole but in those patients who have been observed to develop cardiac arrest suggest that ventricular fibrillation is nearly always the cause and it may not be preceded by any other form of rhythm or conduction disorder.

Although the final mechanism of death may be ventricular fibrillation in the majority of cases, this does not necessarily imply that the same circumstances are always responsible for this arrhythmia. The observations of Wit and others (19) suggest that instantaneous or near instantaneous death may well be due to re-entry within ischaemic myocardium. This form of ventricular fibrillation may be prevented specifically by pre-treatment with beta-adrenergic blocking drugs or a calcium blocker. At a later stage of infarction, ischaemic Purkinje fibres may be the cause of ventricular fibrillation or the basis of enhanced automaticity. Such activity might most appropriately be prevented by sodium blocking drugs such as lignocaine, procainamide or mexiletine.

Risk Factors and Sudden Death
Considerable attention has been paid to the question as to whether sudden death victims differ from those who die less suddenly from myocardial infarction and from those with non-fatal myocardial infarction.

In looking at the conventional risk factors, such as serum cholesterol, systolic blood pressure and cigarette smoking, Kannel et al. (2) reported no appreciable difference between the victims of sudden death and those having a myocardial infarction. Similar findings have been reported by others (20, 21) but Hinkel et al. (22) have suggested that both alcohol and cigarettes are particularly associated with sudden death.

In studies conducted in New York (20) sudden death (defined as death in 48 hours) was found particularly commonly in the physically least active group, especially if they indulged in smoking. Evidence from Morris et al. (23) also suggested that those who indulged in habitual leisure-time physical activity were less likely to have rapidly fatal heart attacks. By contrast, Punsar and Karvonen (24) found that initially healthy lumberjacks, doing work requiring more energy than any other occupation, had an exceptionally high incidence of coronary heart disease; it was recognised, however, that these men had other major risk factors. Wilhelmsen et al. (25) showed that low physical activity during leisure-time but not during work was a risk factor. These authors point out the complex relationship involved. Thus, they found that those who were physically active in their occupation were more often smokers, whereas those who were physically active during leisure-time were more often non-smokers. Furthermore, the same relationships were found with respect to alcoholic intemperance.

A relationship between the Type A personality and sudden death has been suggested by Freidman and Rosenman (26) but this lacks confirmation.

Anderson et al. (27) have claimed that the excess of death in soft-water areas is entirely accounted for by an increased incidence of sudden death.

Although this review is concerned primarily with the detection of risk in apparently healthy persons, it is important to realise that there are many cases of unrecognised angina in the community whose identification might permit the administration of prophylactic measures. However, Rose et al. (28), using a standardised questionnaire, showed that angina, which was present in 5 per cent of the population studied, predicted only one-fifth of the coronary heart disease deaths in the succeeding 5 years. The predictive value of combining angina with ECG abnormalities ("suspect ischaemia") proved much better. In men aged 50 - 59, the 17 per cent of those screened who were found to have "suspect ischaemia" yielded 51 per cent of all the 5 year coronary heart disease deaths.

It is possible that the best predictor of sudden death would be the state of the coronary arteries and of the myocardium, as demonstrated by coronary arteriography and left ventriculography. However, it is unrealistic to consider these potentially hazardous investigations for screening the asymptomatic, although it may have an important prognostic function in those with symptoms or with ECG abnormalities.

Much attention has been devoted to the question as to whether ventricular premature beats are an indicator of a liability to sudden death. This view has been reinforced by an increasing body of evidence that in patients who have recovered from infarction, the demonstration of the more severe types of ventricular arrhythmia appears to be a good predictor of sudden death within the next few months (29 - 31). However, it is becoming increasingly clear that this relationship concerns particularly the survivors of myocardial infarction; even then it probably only applies when the ventricular arrhythmias are associated with significant myocardial damage (32).

The prognostic significance of ventricular premature beats in patients without manifest coronary disease is less convincing. Thus, although a relationship between ventricular arrhythmias and sudden death is apparent in Hinkle's study (22), the association between ventricular arrhythmias and subsequent death was virtually confined to those who already had manifestations of coronary arterial disease. In the study of Reid et al. (33) ventricular premature beats were rare and poor predictors of subsequent death.

In the community heart disease study undertaken in Tecumseh (34), it was noted that ventricular premature contractions were prognostically significant and that the frequency of ventricular premature contractions in addition to the presence of intraventricular conduction defects predicted 38 of 45 sudden deaths that occurred. However, more detailed analysis of the results showed that the high incidence of sudden death in those with ventricular premature beats was virtually confined to patients over the age of 70 and/or those with pre-existing coronary arterial disease. There was only one sudden death in a patient with ventricular premature beats who was less than 70 without known heart disease.

In the Seven Countries Study (35) a crude relationship was found between ventricular premature beats and coronary heart disease, but this became weak when age, blood pressure and other coronary risks cause were accounted for.

Blackburn et al. (36) in a review of this subject concluded "that there is no significant independent predictive information in ventricular premature beats at rest or induced by exercise for coronary disease risk in middle-aged men clinically free of coronary disease". They consider that "intervention on ventricular premature beats is unlikely to have a powerful effect on the frequency of sudden coronary death in persons at high risk due to primary coronary risk factors".

Premonitory Symptoms

There has been considerable interest in the possibility of identifying "prodromal symptoms" of sudden death. Many studies (5, 37 - 40) have shown that myocardial infarction is preceded in about 60 - 70 per cent of cases by the recent onset or worsening of the pre-existing angina and in many other cases by rather more non-specific symptoms such as fatigue and dyspnoea. It is clearly more difficult to know whether victims of sudden death have had prodromal symptoms. However, Kuller, Cooper and Perper (3) reported that 38 per cent of patients dying suddenly in Baltimore had seen a physician in the preceding two weeks. Fulton et al. (40) in a community study in Edinburgh of 25,000 middle-aged males reported that 40 per cent of those dying suddenly had seen their general practitioner within four weeks of death. In both Baltimore and Edinburgh a high proportion of patients who attended their doctor did so not because of any identifiable prodromal symptoms but for such reasons as routine check-ups, repeat prescriptions, indigestion and influenza. Only 10 (12 per cent) of 87 patients dying suddenly in Edinburgh had consulted their doctor because of new or worsening anginal pain compared with 34 (33 per cent) of 104 patients who proceeded to an infarction. By contrast, in the Imminent Myocardial Infarction Rotterdam Study (41), 19 (31 per cent) of 62 sudden death victims had reported "prodromal" symptoms, but they constituted only 1.5 per cent of those with such symptoms. It was of interest in the Baltimore studies that the complaint of chest pain as a prodromal symptom was twice as common in those with a history of heart disease who died suddenly as it was in those who had no such history.

Unusual fatigue has been particularly highlighted as an important premonitory symptom. Thus, in the studies of Kuller et al. (3) this symptom was present in 79 per cent of those with a history of heart disease who proceeded to sudden death, although the incidence was only 35 per cent in those without a preceding history of heart disease. Furthermore, "unusual fatigue" was experienced in 13 - 20 per cent of living controls. If we apply these figures to the Edinburgh community of 25,000 middle-aged patients, 19 of previously heart disease-free individuals would have this symptom as a prodrome of sudden death compared with some 4,000 individuals in the same community having this symptom without doing so. Such symptoms as shortness of breath, palpitation and over-work are even less discriminatory.

Precipitating Events

Controversy continues as to whether psychological or physical stress are common precipitators of sudden death. Certainly, the occasional dramatic story lends circumstantial evidence. Rahe et al. (42) observed that there was marked elevation in life change just six months prior to infarction or death, compared with the same time interval one year earlier. This elevation was particularly apparent in sudden death victims. Myers and Dewar (43) reported that psychological stress had occurred in the preceding 30 minutes in 23 per cent of coronary heart disease deaths coming to the Coroner, as compared with 8 per cent of patients with non-fatal myocardial infarction. In the study of Kuller et al. (3) from Baltimore, 13 per cent of surviving myocardial infarction patients and 14 per cent of sudden deaths were identified as having a possible acute precipitating event in close proximity to the onset. However, these authors point out that it is very difficult to determine the frequency of such events in a general population.

Similarly, there appears to be the occasional clear relationship to physical effort. Sudden death has been attributed to snow shovelling (44), exercise tests and training programmes (45). Friedman et al. (46) have reported that 37 per cent of individuals dying instantaneously had been undertaking strenuous activity shortly beforehand, but the amount of exercise was not unusual for those concerned. It may be concluded that strenuous physical exertion is a rare precipitant of sudden death.

It has been pointed out by Wikland (47) and by Kuller et al. (3) that the majority of sudden deaths occur at home. Myers and Dewar (43) found that individuals dying suddenly had often been active around the house prior to this event and that disproportionately few actually "died in their sleep". A similar observation was made by Friedman et al. (46).

Myers and Dewar (43) also commented on the frequency with which sudden death followed upon a meal accompanied by a large amount of alcohol. They failed to find a relationship between the actual smoking of a cigarette and sudden death.

Other environmental precipitants may include high ambient carbon monoxide levels (48) and extremes in temperature (49).

Infection as a precipitant of sudden death in patients with coronary arterial disease has been little investigated; a recent report by Nicholls and Thomas (50) on a high incidence of Coxsackie infection in patients with acute myocardial infarction has drawn attention to its possible role.

Summary
Fifteen to 25 per cent of all sudden deaths occur in individuals who have not been known to have previous symptoms of coronary heart disease. It is probable that most of them have hearts "too good to die" and their identification is therefore of great importance. However, it does not seem that any risk factors, premonitory symptoms or other characteristics enable us to identify many such patients in advance. At present, the prevention of sudden death must depend upon community wide measures to control the main risk factors and the availability of rapid retrieval systems, where possible.

REFERENCES

(1) Mathewson, F.A.L., Brereton, C.C., Keltie, W.A. and Paul, G.I. (1965): Can. Med. Ass. J., 92, 947.
(2) Kannel, W.B., Doyle, J.T., McNamara, P.M., Quickenton, P. and Gordon, T. (1975): Circulation, 51, 606.
(3) Kuller, L.H., Perper, J.A. and Cooper, M.C. (1975): Sudden and unexpected death due to arteriosclerotic heart disease. In Modern Trends in Cardiology, 3rd Ed. Ed. Oliver, M.F. Butterworth, London, p. 292.
(4) Pell, S. and D'Alonzo, C.A. (1964): New Engl. J. Med., 270, 915.
(5) Armstrong, A., Duncan, B., Oliver, M.F., Julian, D.G., Donald, K.W., Fulton, M., Lutz, W. and Morrison, S.L. (1972): Brit. Heart J., 34, 67.
(6) Cobb, L.A., Baum, R.S., Alvarez, H. and Schaffer, W.A. (1975): Circulation, 51-52 (Suppl. III), 223.
(7) Weaver, W.D., Lorch, G.S., Alvarez, H.A. and Cobb, L.A. (1976): Circulation, 54, 895.
(8) Spain, D.M. and Bradess, V.A. (1960): Amer. J. Med. Sci., 240, 701.
(9) Spain, D.M. and Bradess, V.A. (1960): Circulation, 22, 816 (Abstract).
(10) Roberts, W.C. and Buja, L.M. (1972): Amer. J. Med., 52, 425.
(11) Adelson, L. and Hoffman, W. (1961): J.A.M.A., 176, 129.
(12) Chahine, R.A. and Luchi, R.J. (1976): Amer. J. Cardiol., 37, 936.
(13) Lewis, A.J., Burchell, H.B. and Titus, J.L. (1969): Amer. J. Cardiol., 23, 43.
(14) Sugiura, M. and Okada, R. (1970): Geriatrics, 25, 130.
(15) Edwards, J.E. (1971): Prog. Cardiovasc. Dis., 13, 309.
(16) Naeim, F., De le Maza, L.M. and Robbins, S.L. (1972): Circulation, 45, 1231.
(17) Pantridge, J.F. and Geddes, J.S. (1967): Lancet, 2, 271.
(18) Cobb, L.A., Conn, R.D., Sanson, W.E. and Philbin, J.E. (1971): Circulation, 43 (Suppl. II), 139.

(19) Bigger, J.T. Dresdale, R.J., Heissenbuttel, R.H., Weld, F.M. and Wit, A.L. (1977): Prog. Cardiovasc. Dis., 19, 255.
(20) Shapiro, S., Weinblatt, E., Frank, C.W. and Sagan, R.V. (1969): Amer. J. Publ. Hlth., 59 (Suppl. 2), 1.
(21) Stamler, J. (1975): Circulation, 52 (Suppl. III), 258.
(22) Hinkle, L.E., Carven, S.T. and Stevens, M. (1969): Amer. J. Cardiol., 24, 629.
(23) Morris, J.N., Chave, S.P.W., Adam, C., Sirey, C., Epstein, L. and Sheehan, D.J. (1973): Lancet, 1, 333.
(24) Punsar, S. and Karvonen, M.J. (1976): In Physical Activity and Coronary Disease. Eds. Manninen, V. and Halonen, P.I. Advances in Cardiology, S. Karger Basel, 18, 196.
(25) Wilhelmsen, L., Tibblin, G., Aurell, M., Bjure, J., Ekström-Jodal, B. and Grimby, G. (1976): In Physical Activity and Coronary Disease. Eds. Manninen, V. and Halonen, P.I. Advances in Cardiology, S. Karger Basel, 18, 217.
(26) Friedman, M. and Rosenman, R.H. (1959): J.A.M.A., 169, 1286.
(27) Anderson, T.W., Le Riche, W.N. and McKay, J.S. (1969): New Engl. J. Med., 280, 805.
(28) Rose, G., Reid, D.D., Hamilton, P.J.S., McCartney, P., Keen, H. and Jarrett, R.J. (1977): Lancet, 1, 105.
(29) Kotler, M.N., Tabatznik, B., Mower, M.M. and Tominaga, S. (1973): Circulation, 47, 959.
(30) Vismara, L.A., Amsterdam, E.A. and Mason, D.T. (1975): Amer. J. Med., 59, 6.
(31) Moss, A.J., De Camilla, J., Mietlowski, W., Greene, W.A., Goldstein, S. and Locksley, R. (1975): Circulation, 52 (Suppl. III), 204.
(32) Schulze, R.A., Strauss, H.W. and Pitt, B. (1977): Amer. J. Med., 62, 192.
(33) Reid, D.D., Brett, G.Z., Hamilton, P.J.S., Jarrett, R.J., Keen, H. and Rose, G. (1974): Lancet, 1, 469.
(34) Chiang, B.N., Perlman, L.V., Fulton, M., Ostrander, L.D. and Epstein, F.H. (1970): Circulation, 41, 31.
(35) Keys, A. (1970): Circulation, 41 (Suppl. I).
(36) Blackburn, H., DeBacker, G., Crow, R., Prineas, R. and Jacobs, D. (1976): In Physical Activity and Coronary Disease. Eds. Manninen, V. and Halonen, P.I. Advances in Cardiology, S. Karger Basel, 18, 208.
(37) Solomon, H.A., Edwards, A.L. and Killip, T. (1969): Circulation, 40, 463.
(38) Stowers, M. and Short, D. (1970): Brit. Heart J., 32, 833.
(39) Feinleib, M., Simon, A.B., Gillum, F. and Margolis, J.R. (1975): Circulation, 51-52 (Suppl. III), 155.
(40) Fulton, M., Lutz, W., Donald, K.W., Kirby, B.J., Duncan, G., Morrison, S.L., Kerr, F., Julian, D.G. and Oliver, M.F. (1972): Lancet, 1, 860.
(41) Lubsen, J., Pool, J. and Van den Does, E. (1976): Hart Bulletin, 7, 114.
(42) Rahe, R.H., Romo, M., Bennett, L. and Siltonen, P. (1974): Arch. Intern. Med., 133, 221.
(43) Myers, A. and Dewar, H.A. (1975): Brit. Heart J., 37, 1133.
(44) Burgess, A.M. (1965): Rhode Island Med. J., 48, 131.
(45) Cantwell, J.D. and Fletcher, G.F. (1969): J.A.M.A., 210, 130.
(46) Friedman, M., Mainwaring, J.H., Rosenman, R.H., Donlon, G., Ortega, P. and Grube, S.M. (1973): J.A.M.A., 225, 1319.
(47) Wikland, B. (1971): Acta Med. Scand. Suppl. 524.
(48) Goldsmith, J.R. and Landaw, S.A. (1968): Science, 162, 1352.
(49) Protos, A.A., Caracta, A. and Gross, L. (1971): J. Amer. Geriat. Soc., 19, 526.
(50) Nicholls, A.C. and Thomas, M. (1977): Lancet, 1, 883.

QUESTIONS

Dr. D. Krikler asked whether some cases of sudden death attributed to coronary
disease, but in whom there was no evidence of this at autopsy, were not better
classified as "sudden cardiac death"; perhaps a search should be made in resuscitated survivors for evidence of Q-T prolongation syndromes and other possible
non-coronary factors. Dr. Robert Bruce stressed the importance of the summation
of various known indices of risk in patients with sudden death during exercise
programmes, or exercise tests, and instanced one case of inherent Q-T prolongation
syndrome that had been aggravated by quinidine. Dr. Koen Bruyneel asked whether
sudden death was more common in those with high intelligence quotients; Dr. Julian
did not feel that there was any good evidence to support this. Dr. Lawson McDonald
stressed the importance of the definition of "sudden death", which could cover
different meanings in terms of time periods in different series; Dr. Julian agreed
that precise definition was essential.

IMPLICATIONS OF REGIONAL CARDIAC MECHANICAL FUNCTION IN MYOCARDIAL ISCHEMIA AND
INFARCTION - A STRATEGY FOR PRESYMPTOMATIC DETECTION

Jeremy Swan

Cedars-Sinai Medical Centre, Los Angeles, California, U.S.A.

Myocardial ischemia is the direct cause of the clinical manifestations of coronary
heart disease and myocardial infarction. For practical clinical purposes, the necessary antecedent condition for production of ischemia is limitation of blood flow
caused by the increased resistance of coronary arteries partially occluded due to
atherosclerosis, or less commonly, by coronary spasm, embolus or spontaneous thrombosis. Certain other clinical syndromes including certain myopathies and Barlow's
syndrome may also cause ischemia. Given a pre-existing "anatomic" limitation to
myocardial oxygen supply, clinical manifestations of ischemic heart disease often
first become apparent during a "physiologic" increase in myocardial oxygen demand.
When this imbalance between regional myocardial oxygen supply is sufficiently severe,
as with complete cessation of regional blood flow, the first irreversible changes in
myocardial cells begin to appear at about 20 minutes (1). Lesser reduction of regional blood flow result in a longer duration of myocardial survival and a smaller
territory of involvement.

The interrelation between blood flow, oxygen demand and the manifestations of ischemia is complex. A moderate degree of blood flow reduction may be well tolerated by
the cardiac muscle, because it is sufficient for resting metabolic needs. The bio-
logic and clinical manifestations of cardiac ischemia then develop when myocardial
work is increased, as during physical activity or endogenous cardiac stimulation.
The development of the first recognizable manifestations of cardiac ischemia, however, is generally not accompanied by clinical symptoms. As the factors controlling
the relationship between regional myocardial oxygen supply and demand move the equation toward further imbalance (Figure 1), the familiar clinical markers of cardiac
ischemia, namely angina pectoris, or less commonly, dyspnea and fatigue.

It is now clear that angina pectoris and acute myocardial infarction - the classic
clinical markers of ischemic heart disease - develop at a relatively late stage in
the course of cardiac ischemia, and are generally preceded by reproducible changes
in cardiac mechanics. The identification and the significance of altered segmental
myocardial wall motion in detection and evaluation of patients with ischemic heart
disease is the subject of this communication.

Cardiac Mechanics in Ischemia
Although the work of Tennant and Wiggers (2) in 1933 is generally accepted as the
first serious study of the changes of mechanical function of the heart associated
with coronary occlusion, Sir Thomas Lewis (3) wrote a clear graphic description of
the course of events following ligation of a coronary artery a quarter of a century
previously. He noted an immediate change in epicardial colour upon ligation of a
coronary artery. "Within a few minutes the damaged ventricular muscle dilates and
is ballooned. With each systole of the heart it becomes more swollen until eventually no visible contraction is present". In the past decade, detailed experimental
studies on the nature and time course of mechanical, biochemical, electrical and
hemodynamic changes consequent on occlusion of a single coronary artery have been
extensively reported (4 - 7). Changes in systemic hemodynamics are related predominantly to the extent of territory supplied by the occluded vessel or vessels. Reduction of coronary blood supply to all portions of the heart equally, or reduction

in oxygen content of coronary blood results in almost immediate global reduction in the force of cardiac contraction with a consequent increase in diastolic left ventricular pressure, reduction in arterial blood pressure, and a reduction in total cardiac output (5). In contrast, when blood flowing through a branch of a coronary vessel is importantly reduced, little if any alteration in diastolic ventricular pressure, cardiac output and blood pressure occur despite absence of contraction in the underperfused segment itself. Thus, in addition to being undetectible clinically, regional myocardial ischemia may also not be apparent from global measurements of cardiac performance.

To study regional mechanics, a number of gauges have been developed which allow assessment of regional function during the induction of regional ischemia (8). Figure 2 shows that as regional coronary perfusion was reduced in stepwise fashion, regional function initially decreased minimally until coronary perfusion pressure reached 50 - 65 mmHg and regional coronary blood flow was approximately 60% of control (Figure 3). When pressure and flow were reduced below these critical ranges, however regional function decreased sharply (9). There is a specific sequence of changes in the pattern of wall motion with ischemia which can be observed during this procedure, or seen in a contracted time course in a region rendered acutely ischemic by total occlusion (Figure 3) (10). The segment first begins to lengthen in late systole. This lengthening occurs at a progressively earlier point in systole until there is little or no shortening during systole. These changes represent a progressive decrease in the capacity of ischemia of the muscle segment to shorten during systole against the stresses developed by the contraction of normally perfused segments of the left ventricle. In this regard, plots of left ventricular pressure against segment length invariably shows four morphological patterns (11) (Figure 4) which relate directly to specific left ventricular contraction patterns as described by Herman (12) in man. Reoxygenation following occlusions of short duration, revealed a return to normal pattern in the reverse order of development. With partial occlusion, or in the early stages (less than 30 minutes) of a complete occlusion, the apparently noncontractile myocardium remains responsive to interpolated extra systoles or to intra-arterial injection of calcium. However, if occlusion is prolonged, permanent changes occur in the ischemic area. Function is not restored by reperfusion nor are such muscle segments any longer responsive to otherwise effective stimuli, representing the physiological and functional evidence of myocardial cell death.

The relation between these changes in regional performance and global left ventricular function also has been determined in the experimental animal. The first identifiable abnormality of global left ventricular function was a small decrease in peak negative dp/dt, which occurs concomitant with, or just after regional lactate production and reduction in segmental myocardial function (13). These changes are usually first identifiable with a reduction in coronary arterial flow to approximately 50% of the control value. Epicardial ST segment abnormalities over the ischemic zone usually cannot be detected until coronary flow is further reduced.

Taken together, this experimental evidence defines a hierarchy of changes which accompany reduction in regional coronary blood flow. Alteration in cardiac mechanics is the first readily detectable change and is closely associated with an abnormality of regional metabolism. This is followed later by changes in the electrocardiographic ST segment and only after a large mass of myocardium is affected does global ventricular performance become detectably altered.

Relevant Studies in Man
Although controlled studies are more difficult to obtain in the human, the likelihood appears strong that this hierarchy of markers of cardiac ischemia are similar to those defined in the experimental animal. Two sets of patient studies appear to be relevant to this judgement. In patients with preinfarction angina, but without

cardiac pain or electrocardiographic changes at the time of cardiac catheterization, variable and frequently large areas of dyskinesis can be observed angiographically (14) even in the absence of symptoms or ECG changes. In addition, coronary artery disease patients with normal LV contraction patterns at rest develop reversible dyskinetic patterns during cardiac pacing, hand grip dynamometry, or catecholamine infusion. Regional dyskinesia in such patients may or may not be associated with abnormal lactate production, and when lactate production does appear, it develops before changes of the electrocardiogram or the recognition of angina by the subject patient (15). The second set of data comes from patients undergoing surgical re-vascularization. Following surgery, areas of dyskinesis often become normal, and the end-diastolic pressure falls to normal values. Revascularization also has been shown to negate the ischemic consequences of cardiac pacing, including restoration of normal lactate metabolism (16). Taken together with the animal data, therefore, these data imply that a hierarchy of recognizable manifestations of ischemia exists, that these markers precede clinical signs, and that like overt symptoms, they can be induced by stress and relieved by therapeutic measures. As a corollary, the presence of symptoms, particularly if dyspnea and fatigue are present, suggests the presence of relatively severe regional ischemia.

Non-invasive Demonstration of Regional Dysfunction in Man

Although selective left ventriculography is currently the method of choice for demonstration of abnormal cardiac mechanical function, its disadvantages are obvious. First, it is an invasive procedure which carries significant morbidity in addition to a small but real mortality. Second, the procedure is not without discomfort, both physical and emotional, to the subject patient. These factors, plus the cost in capital investment and operational expenses, limits its use to a very small segment of the population. For these reasons, regional cardiac performance must be evaluated by non-invasive procedures in order to have wide applicability.

There are currently at least three techniques which hold substantial promise. Although like contrast angiography, each has advantages and disadvantages, it seems likely that all will find a role in clinical diagnosis.

Radioisotopes can be used in a manner similar to radiological angiography to visualize the right and left heart during cardiac contraction, with a degree of detail which approaches but is not yet equal to that of conventional angiography (17). This technique has recently been used to identify the development of an abnormal regional contraction pattern after exercise (18). Nuclear techniques are likely to remain expensive both in the capital investment required for the necessary cameras and computational devices and in the cost of isotopes for repeated procedures. Thus, these techniques will be restricted to use by a Department of Nuclear Medicine, and widespread utilization will be sharply limited by the number of qualified physicians and technologists to perform appropriate studies.

Ultrasonography can also be used to provide important information concerning regional wall function (Figure 5). The most promising option available are the "sector scanners", which reduced the limitations imposed by conventional M Mode echocardiography, which can visualize only a single point on the ventricular wall (19). Sector scanners simultaneously recorded a number of M Mode images, and the output is then displayed in a format comparable to conventional angiography. The ability of these devices to record wall motion with sufficient resolution to permit precise analysis of segmental wall motion remains to be clearly demonstrated (20).

The cardiokymograph is a simple magnetic field generator, the output of which is perturbated by the movement of tissue immediately (2 - 3 cm) beneath it (2). Perturbation of the generated electromagnetic field is identified by a balancing circuit and displayed as an analog signal. Current experience in our clinical and animal laboratories suggest a useful role for this device in the identification of abnormal contraction of myocardial segments (22). In fact, this device has certain highly desirable characteristics for the early practical detection of presymptomatic cardiac ischemia. Comparative studies in dogs have indicated that the output from the CKG is remarkably similar to that of the length gauge sutured to the beating heart (23), and that coronary occlusion results in essentially identical changes in the output of both devices. When placed over the anterior chest wall of man, the CKG output is thought to represent the anterior left ventricular wall (Figure 6). As in experimental cardiac ischemia in the dog, a series of changes in this pattern can be observed to occur in the presence of regional cardiac ischemia in man. Late systolic changes are the first deviation from the normal followed by mid, early and pan systolic outward motion. In exercise studies in man (Figure 7), the development of abnormalities at the end of a standard exercise test are highly correlated with the presence of coronary artery disease (24), and these abnormalities are only rarely observed to develop in individuals with normal coronary arteries. At present therefore, the sensitivity of the CKG appear to exceed that of the ST segment of the stress electrocardiogram, and its specificity appears to be at least comparable.

The particular merit of the CKG is its low cost, portability and ease of application. The head itself weighs a few ounces, and the controlling device and analog recorder a few pounds. The ECG and other non-invasive recordings are recorded simultaneously, thus, the CKG may be placed in strategically important clinical locations and in a practicing physician's office. It is therefore quite applicable as a screening tool in a wide variety of circumstances. However, the basic nature of the signal is complex and interpretation is currently justified largely by empiric application.

Summary
Alteration in regional cardiac mechanics is probably the earliest readily recordable evidence of cardiac ischemia secondary to coronary artery disease or other causes, and clearly precedes clinical symptoms. Early in its course of development, coronary heart disease is characterized by the development of ischemic manifestations when the factors that control the myocardial oxygen supply-demand ratio are altered. Thus, the demonstration of regional myocardial ischemia with stress allows for detection of ischemic heart disease prior to symptoms, with a high degree of suspicion in the presence of an important coronary obstruction. Such presymptomatic detection of patients with covert coronary artery disease is dependent on non-invasive procedures. Preferably such procedures are based on simple technology and can be employed by non-physicians.

The detection of presymptomatic coronary artery disease is desirable to better define the natural history of this disease and to identify these cohorts of individuals who can be shown to be at unusually high risk. These subsets would then be the natural targets for the various measures of primary and secondary prevention of adverse coronary events, and would provide a far more suitable population for the rational employment of clinical trials of a wide variety of therapeutic interventions. Finally, the simple identification of an asymptomatic population in which the prevalence of coronary heart disease was several times that of the normal asymptomatic population would render epidemological studies more likely to result in definitive answers over a shorter time span and a fraction of the cost of similar studies of total populations.

REFERENCES

(1) Jennings, R.B. and Ganote, C.E. (1974): Circulat. Res., 35, Suppl. 3, 156.
(2) Tennant, R. and Wiggers, C.J. (1935): Amer. J. Physiol., 112, 351.
(3) Lewis, T., Sir (1909): Heart, 1, 98.
(4) Theroux, P., Franklin, D., Ross, J., Jr. and Kemper, W.S. (1974): Circulat. Res., 35, 896.
(5) Apstein, C.S., Deckelbaum, L., Mueller, M., Hagopian, L. and Hood, W.B., Jr.

(1977): Circulation, 55, 864.

(6) Kjekshus, J.K., Maroko, P.R. and Sobel, B.E. (1972): Cardiovasc. Res., 6, 490.

(7) Owen, P., Thomas, M., Young, V. and Opie, L. (1970): Amer. J. Cardiol., 25, 562.

(8) Forrester, J.S., Tyberg, J.V., Wyatt, H.L., Goldner, S., Parmley, W.W. and Swan, H.J.C. (1974): J. Appl. Physiol., 37, 771.

(9) Wyatt, H.L., Forrester, J.S., Tyberg, J.V., Goldner, S., Logan, S.E., Parmley, W.W. and Swan, H.J.C. (1975): Amer. J. Cardiol., 36, 185.

(10) Forrester, J.S., Wyatt, H.L., da Luz, P.L., Tyberg, J.V., Diamond, G.A. and Swan, H.J.C. (1976): Circulation, 54, 64.

(11) Waters, D.D., Forrester, J.S. and Swan, H.J.C.: Detection and quantification of myocardial ischemia. Submitted to Annals of Internal Medicine. (In press).

(12) Herman, M.V., Heinle, R.A., Klein, R.A. and Gorlin, R. (1967): N. Engl. J. Med., 277, 222.

(13) Waters, D.D., da Luz, P.L., Wyatt, H.L., Swan, H.J.C. and Forrester, J.S. (1977): Amer. J. Cardiol., 39, 537.

(14) Chatterjee, K., Swan, H.J.C., Parmley, W.W., Sustaita, H., Marcus, H. and Matloff, J. (1972): N. Engl. J. Med., 286, 1117.

(15) Klocke, F.J. and Wittenberg, S.M. (1969): Amer. J. Cardiol., 24, 782.

(16) Dwyer, E.M., Jr., Dell, R.B. and Cannon, P.J. (1973): Circulation, 48, 924.

(17) Zaret, B.L. (1976): Circulation, 53, Suppl. 1, 126.

(18) Berman, D.S., Amsterdam, E.A., Hines, H.H., Salel, A.F., Bailey, G.J., Denardo, G.L. and Mason, D.T. (1977): Amer. J. Cardiol., 39, 341.

(19) Kerber, R.E. and Abboud, F.M. (1973): Circulation, 47, 997.

(20) Von Ramm, T. and Thurstone, F.L. (1976): Circulation, 53, 258.

(21) Vas, R., Joyner, C.R., Pittman, D.E. and Gay, T.C. (1976): IEEE Trans. Biomed. Eng., 23, 49.

(22) Diamond, G.A., Chag, M., Vas, R. et al.: Cardiokymography - Quantitative analysis of regional ischemic left ventricular dysfunction. Amer. J. Cardiol. (In press).

(23) Vas, R., Diamond, G.A., Wyatt, H.L., da Luz, P.L., Swan, H.J.C. and Forrester, J.S.: Noninvasive analysis of regional myocardial wall motion: Cardiokymography. Amer. J. Physiol. (In press).

(24) Forrester, J.S., Vas, R., Diamond, G.A. et al.: Cardiokymography - a new method for assessing segmental wall motion in man. In, Advances in Cardiol. (In press).

QUESTIONS

Dr. Bruce Kottke felt that this technique could be used to show the impaired cardiac function immediately after coronary bypass surgery. Dr. Dennis Krikler raised the question of the detection of anterior wall movement in the case of postero-inferior infarction and wondered about the specificity of the method for localized regional dysfunction: Dr. Swan suggested that additional anterior involvement might be responsible, or alternatively that one would see rotation of the heart because of the infarct. Professor John Shillingford wondered what the instrument was measuring and raised the possibility that the transducer was responding to iron in the blood and myocardium.

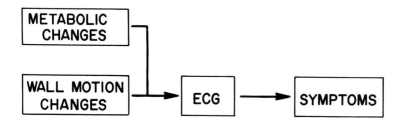

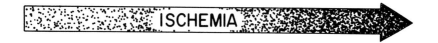

FIG. 1   The hierarchy of changes with increasingly severe ischemia. Recent research indicates that the first detectable changes in parameters of regional
myocardial performance are those of metabolism and segmental wall motion.
As ischemia becomes more severe, electrocardiographic ST-T wave changes
become manifest. Only when regional ischemia becomes severe do symptoms
result.

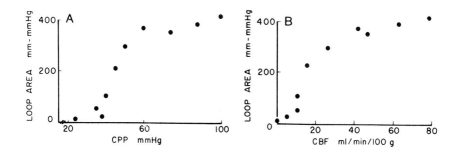

FIG. 2   The relationship between regional myocardial function, as measured by loop
area, and coronary blood flow (CBF) and coronary perfusion pressure (CPP).
As coronary blood flow is progressively reduced to approximately 50% of
control, there is little change in regional myocardial performance. Beyond
this point, there are substantial decrement in function with even minimal
reduction in flow or perfusion pressure.

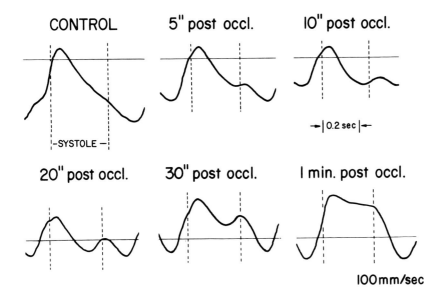

CONTROL 5" post occl. 10" post occl.

-SYSTOLE-

→|0.2 sec|←

20" post occl. 30" post occl. 1 min. post occl.

100mm/sec

FIG. 3   Progressive changes in regional myocardial wall motion following coronary
occlusion, as measured by a length gauge sutured to the epicardial surface
of the left ventricle. Dotted lines represent systole. During the control
state, there is shortening throughout the systole. At five seconds following occlusion, the magnitude of shortening has diminished and a late systolic bulge appears. This bulge progressively encroaches upon shortening in
systole, until by 30 seconds, an M shaped pattern of movement in systole
is apparent. By one minute following occlusion, there is little if any
shortening during the systole. With release of coronary occlusion, segmental wall motion returns to normal in an opposite sequence.

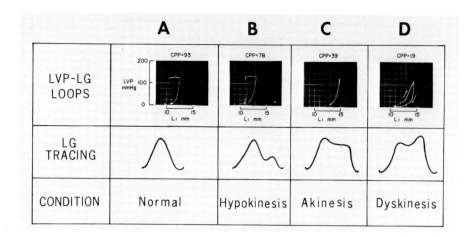

	A	B	C	D
LVP-LG LOOPS	CPP=93	CPP=78	CPP=39	CPP=19
LG TRACING				
CONDITION	Normal	Hypokinesis	Akinesis	Dyskinesis

FIG. 4   Relationship between assessment of regional function by length gauges and cardiac angiography. The top panels illustrate the relationship between the left ventricular pressure (LVP) and myocardial segment length as a "pressure-length loop" for a single cardiac cycle. At rest, the pressure length loop is inscribed in a counterclockwise fashion and has a rectangular morphology. With reduction in regional perfusion (panel B), the first detectable change is a slight diminution in the magnitude of shortening with a bulge in late systole and isometric relaxation. This change in the morphology of the length gauge tracing and the pressure loop is manifest at ventriculography as dysynchrony and/or hypokinesis. With further reduction in flow (panel C), there is absence of shortening on the length gauge tracing, and no area within the pressure-length loop. This is represented by akinesis at left ventriculography. In panel D is shown the final result of reduction in flow in which lengthening during the period of systolic ejection is observed, with a reversed pressure-length loop. This condition is represented at left ventriculography as dyskinesis.

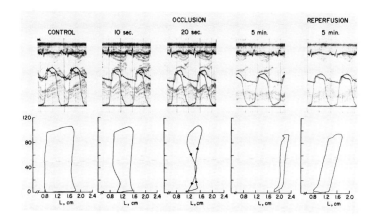

FIG. 5   The echocardiographic representation of altered posterior wall regional
         function following circumflex coronary occlusion in the dog. During the
         control state, there is substantial inward movement recorded by the echo-
         cardiogram and a counterclockwise, rectangular pressure-length loop is ob-
         tained. At ten seconds following coronary occlusion, segment shortening is
         reduced and a late systolic bulge is observed in the pressure-length loop.
         At twenty seconds following occlusion, these changes are more pronounced.
         By five minutes, there is little if any shortening in the posterior wall
         segment. Five minutes following reperfusion, the pressure-length loop has
         returned to a counterclockwise rectangular shape with substantial shorten-
         ing observed during the period of systolic ejection.

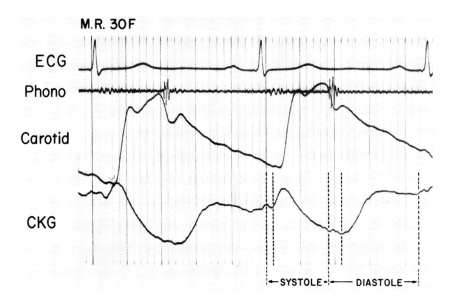

FIG. 6   The normal cardiokymographic tracing at rest, obtained over the V4 position
         on the anterior chest wall. Shown from the top are the electrocardiogram
         (ECG), phonocardiogram (Phono), external carotid pulse wave tracing (Caro-
         tid), and the cardiokymograph tracing (CKG). Dotted lines represent sys-
         tole and diastole. During systolic ejection, there is a smooth inward
         motion recorded by the cardiokymograph. This representation of segmental
         wall motion is strikingly similar to that obtained by a number of other
         invasive devices in both animals and man.

127

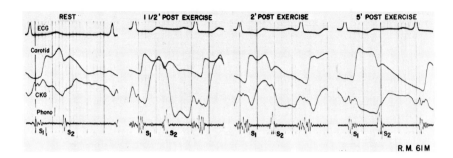

FIG. 7   The effect of exercise upon the cardiokymographic representation of seg-
         mental wall motion in a man with coronary artery disease. Represented on
         the tracings are the electrocardiogram (ECG), carotid pulse tracing (caro-
         tid), cardiokymograph (CKG) and phonocardiogram (phono). At rest, the CKG
         tracing reveals inward movement during the period of systolic ejection. At
         one and one-half minutes following exercise, there is minimal shortening
         during systole ejection, followed by a pronounced outward movement. At two
         minutes following exercise, these changes persist, although diminished in
         magnitude. By five minutes, the CKG tracing has returned to the control
         state.

THE DETECTION OF INCOORDINATE LEFT VENTRICULAR CONTRACTION BY M-MODE ECHOCARDIOGRAPHY

Derek Gibson

Brompton Hospital, London

Abnormalities of mechanical function have been shown to be a sensitive sign of myocardial ischaemia, so that their detection in individual subjects might prove a satisfactory means of detecting early effects of coronary artery disease. At first sight,
M-mode echocardiography might seem an inadequate technique for doing this in view of
the limited region of the cavity that can be studied directly. On the other hand, it
is particularly suited to recording ventricular wall movement since it unequivocally
localizes endo- and epicardial position throughout the cardiac cycle, and because of
its excellent frequency response when a repetition frequency of 1000/sec is used. In
this paper, abnormalities of left ventricular wall movement in patients with documented coronary artery disease will be described, with particular reference to the detection of incoordinate contraction and relaxation. It appears that these abnormalities
may lead to generalized disturbances of left ventricular wall movement even in unaffected regions. These may be detected by M-mode echocardiography even if the primary
abnormality is inaccessible to study.

Standard echocardiographic measurements of left ventricular function are based on two
estimates of cavity size in each cardiac cycle, made at end-systole and end-diastole.
Using a simple computing technique, it is possible to make measurements of wall position and cavity size continuously throughout the cardiac cycle (1). In order to do
this, the echocardiogram is placed on a digitizing table, and a cursor is run along
each of the echoes to be digitized. The position of the cursor is detected electron-
ically, and converted into a series of digital coordinates, up to 100 per cardiac
cycle being generated for each echo and stored in the computer. This process can also
be applied to echoes from the right and left sides of the septum, the anterior cusp
of the mitral valve, and endo- and epicardial surfaces of the septum. It is also
possible to digitize any other continuous signal such as the apexcardiogram or the
left ventricular pressure trace. Once these have been digitized, the computer can
plot them unchanged, or can perform further manipulations on them. For example, the
coordinates of the septum can be subtracted from those of the posterior wall endocardium to derive a continuous measure of dimension, or those of endocardium subtracted from epicardium to derive left ventricular wall thickness. It is also possible to
differentiate a variable with respect to time, so that its rate of change can be calculated. An example of such a plot, taken from a normal subject is shown in Figure 1.
The original information was plotted unchanged in the lowest panel. In the middle is
shown the left ventricular dimension, falling during systole, and increasing rapidly
at first during early diastole, and then more slowly during the period of diastasis.
The timing of aortic valve closure and mitral valve opening are superimposed as two
crosses, defining the period of isovolumic relaxation, and it will be seen that there
has been little change in dimension during this interval. It is also apparent that
mitral valve opening coincides with minimum cavity dimension, suggesting that the
increase during diastole is indeed due to filling. Finally, the top trace gives the
rate of change of dimension, which reaches approximately 10 cm/sec during systole and
20 cm/sec during diastole. These estimates of peak rates of wall movement have been
compared with corresponding measurements from angiogram and satisfactory agreement has
been confirmed (2).

Although these values may give information about a single region of the cavity, they cannot necessarily be extrapolated to the ventricle as a whole if function is incoordinate. The potential significance of this is demonstrated in the echocardiogram shown in Figure 2. The record is taken from a patient who developed a low cardiac output state after open heart surgery. At first sight, ventricular function appears good, with a satisfactory amplitude of posterior wall movement, the small degree of septal movement being common after cardiopulmonary bypass. On closer inspection however, it is apparent that in diastole almost all posterior wall movement occurs before the start of mitral valve opening, and therefore before the onset of left ventricular filling, so that the apparently normal increase in left ventricular dimension occurring during diastole represents no more than a change in left ventricular cavity shape during the period of isovolumic relaxation. Observations such as this suggested that it might be fruitful to study left ventricular wall movement during the two isovolumic periods rather than in filling or ejection. In this way it would be possible to detect non-uniform ventricular function by studying dimension, not in isolation, but in relation to some index of overall function. If left ventricular behaviour is uniform, local and overall function will be in phase with one another, but this close time relation is lost when contraction is incoordinate.

One way to do this is to use the high fidelity left ventricular pressure trace, and to plot the relation between pressure and dimension in the form of a pressure-dimension loop (3). In normal subjects, the shape of the loop is characteristic, and approximates to a rectangle (Figure 3). Four phases can be recognized: isovolumic contraction when pressure rises at constant dimension, ejection when dimension falls at approximately constant pressure, isovolumic relaxation when pressure falls, again at constant pressure, and finally filling when dimension increases at low pressure (4). This rectangular shape has functional significance in that the area of the loop represents stroke work per unit area of myocardium performed on the circulation. The maximum work which could have been performed by the myocardium working over the same range of pressure and dimension is the product of the two, i.e. the area of the rectangle that just encloses the loop. A rectangular loop thus represents the condition of efficient energy transfer from the myocardium to the circulation, and distortion of the loop indicates loss of mechanical efficiency in this process. An example of such a distorted loop is given in Figure 4, from a patient with ischaemic heart disease. It is clear that distortion of the loop results mainly from abnormal wall movement during the two isovolumic periods rather than abnormal pressure changes in ejection or filling.

Unfortunately, measurement of left ventricular pressure directly requires cardiac catheterization, but the timing of the upstroke and the downstroke of the pressure trace can be obtained, with minor delay, from the apexcardiogram (3, 5). This is fortunate, since in clinical left ventricular disease, abnormalities of the loop occur most frequently during the two isovolumic periods. In addition, it is an advantage from the point of view of M-mode echocardiography, that a single regional abnormality of wall motion cannot occur during an isovolumic period. Inward movement in one region of the cavity must be accompanied by equal and opposite net outward movement elsewhere. We have therefore examined the use of simultaneous apex and echocardiogram to detect incoordinate contraction. As with pressure, the results are presented in the form of a loop, which has proved to be rectangular in more than 50 normal subjects studied.(6, Figure 5). The configuration of the loop was abnormal in all of 20 patients with ischaemic heart disease and regional abnormalities of function demonstrable by left ventriculography. The results from one such patient are shown in Figure 6. Although the original plots of wall movement and apexcardiogram appear normal, the time relations between the two, as shown by the loop, are clearly disturbed. During the upstroke of the apexcardiogram, there is an abnormal reduction in dimension. Since this occurs during the period of isovolumic contraction, there must have been outward movement elsewhere, due to delayed onset on contraction in some other region of the ventricle. Similarly, during the downstroke of the apexcardiogram which encompasses the period of isovolumic relaxation, there was a reduction in dimension, suggesting an abnormal increase elsewhere. This indicates that disturbances of wall movement during the isovolumic periods may be of two kinds: either the primary abnormality, or a secondary effect occurring because the volume of blood in the ventricle is constant at these times. During isovolumic contraction, an increase in dimension represents abnormal, and a reduction, normal behaviour, while during isovolumic relaxation, the reverse is the case. The left ventricular angiogram from the same patient is shown in Figure 7, demonstrating an apical area of reduced amplitude of wall movement, well away from the path of the echo beam. By contrast, in Figure 8 is shown the echo dimension apexcardiogram loop from a patient with disease of the right coronary artery, where the disturbances are the opposite of those shown in Figure 6. The corresponding angiogram is reproduced in Figure 9, which demonstrates an inferior aneurysm. Overall experience from 20 patients is shown in the table. This demonstrates that abnormalities of relaxation are commoner than those of contraction, and that of the former, those representing compensatory behaviour appear approximately three times as common as those due to the primary abnormality of wall movement itself.

These and other results suggest that M-mode echocardiography used in this way may be a sensitive means of detecting incoordinate left ventricular contraction due to regional abnormalities of function. Ischaemic heart disease is an important, but by no means the only cause of these. Other clinical associations include congestive or hypertrophic cardiomyopathy, valvular heart disease, particularly when significant left ventricular hypertrophy is present, and hypertension. They may also appear after open heart surgery, due to limitations of the procedure used for myocardial preservation. M-mode echocardiography thus provides a means of detecting such abnormalities in the general population, along with information about cavity size and peak rates of wall movement. Although giving less direct information that two dimensional techniques about the left ventricular cavity, this is compensated for by its ability to detect and quantify minor abnormalities of wall motion.

REFERENCES

(1) Upton, M.T. and Gibson, D.G. (1977): Study of left ventricular function from digitized echocardiograms. Progress in Cardiovascular Diseases. (In press).
(2) Gibson, D.G. and Brown, D.J. (1975): Brit. Heart J., 37, 677.
(3) Gibson, D.G. and Brown, D.J. (1976): Brit. Heart J., 38, 8.
(4) Rushmer, R.F. (1956): Amer. J. Physiol., 186, 115.
(5) Manolas, J., Rutishauser, W., Wirz, P. and Arbenz, U. (1975): Brit. Heart J., 37, 1263.
(6) Venco, A., Gibson, D.G. and Brown, D.J. (1977): Brit. Heart J., 39, 117.

QUESTIONS

Dr. Lawson McDonald asked about the value of ultrasound as a detector of changes in physical characteristics of the myocardium. Dr. Gibson thought that better techniques were required for this purpose but one could already detect fibrosis of the septum; the information needed to be obtained in this way and one might possibly be able to detect the early changes of ischaemia in this way. In response to Dr. Kennedy, he did not think that obstructive airways disease presented a major problem in echocardiography. Dr. Attilio Maseri suggested that changes such as had been described in cardiac ischaemia might persist for some time after the ischaemia had been corrected. Dr. R. Vermeulen thought that the EF slope of the mitral valve was often influenced by the presence of ischaemic heart disease, but Dr. Gibson did not agree. He agreed with Dr. Robert Bruce that the echocardiographic detection of areas of asynchrony could be important in identifying zones where re-entry might arise.

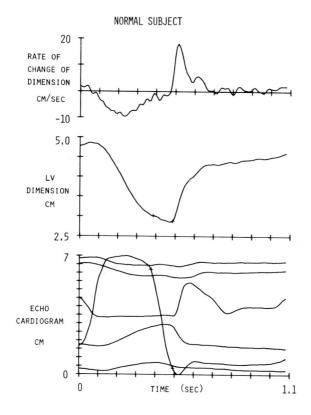

FIG. 1   Digitized left ventricular echocardiogram from a normal subject, with apexcardiogram superimposed. The lowest panel represents the original data,
with crosses indicating the timing of aortic valve closure and mitral valve
opening. The middle panel represents left ventricular dimension and the
top represents rate of change of dimension.

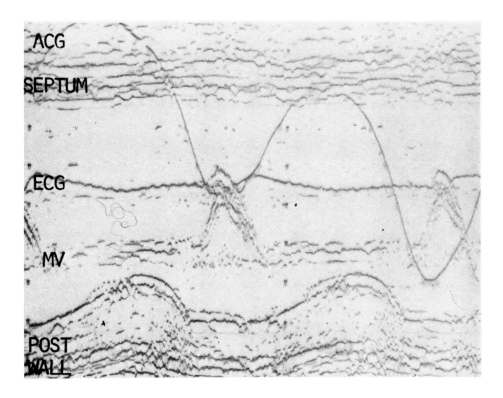

FIG. 2   Echocardiogram of a patient who developed a low cardiac output state after surgery. Outward posterior left ventricular wall movement is almost complete before the start of mitral valve opening.

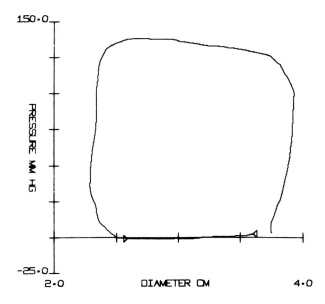

FIG. 3   Pressure-dimension loop from a patient with normal left ventricular function.

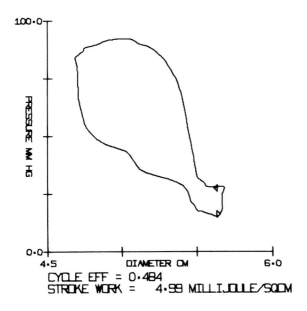

FIG. 4   Pressure-dimension loop from a patient with ischaemic heart disease.

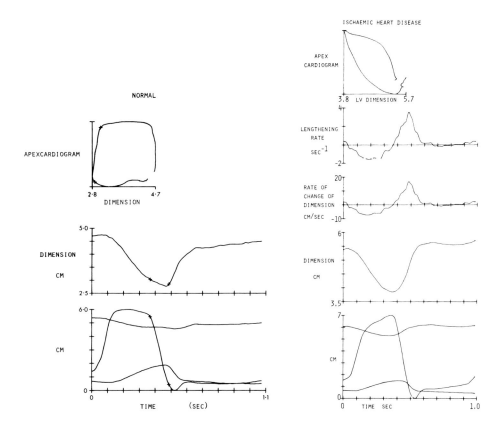

FIG. 5   Computer output of digitized apex and echocardiograms from a normal sub-
         ject showing from below, echoes from septum and posterior wall and the
         apexcardiogram. Above are changes in dimension and (top) the echo dimen-
         sion apexcardiogram loop, which is approximately rectangular.

FIG. 6   Computer output of digitized apex and echocardiograms from a patient with
         ischaemic heart disease. There are abnormal dimension changes during the
         upstroke and downstroke of the apexcardiogram.

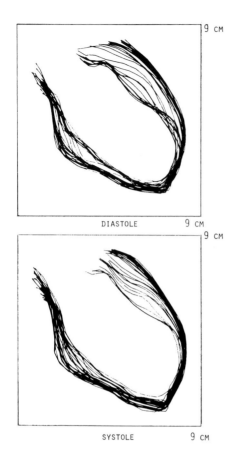

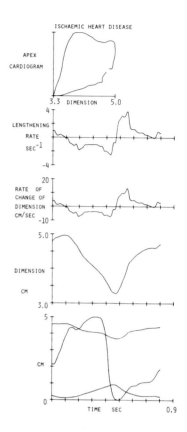

DIASTOLE   9 CM

SYSTOLE   9 CM

FIG. 7   Digitized left ventricular cineangiogram from the same patients as that shown in Figure 6. Cavity outlines of cine frames are shown superimposed. There is an area of apical hypokinesia.

FIG. 8   Computer output of digitized apex and echocardiograms from a patient with ischaemic heart disease and inferior aneurysm.

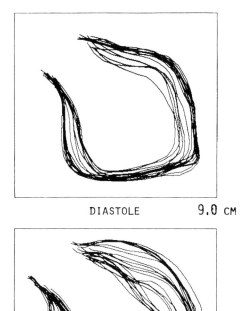

DIASTOLE   9.0 CM

SYSTOLE   9.0 CM

FIG. 9   Digitized cineangiogram from the patient shown in Figure 8.

MYOCARDIAL SCINTIGRAPHY AND RECONSTRUCTIVE TOMOGRAPHIC POSITRON IMAGING USING
NITROGEN-13 LABELLED AMMONIA

Leon Resnekov

University of Chicago, Chicago, U.S.A.

INTRODUCTION

The need for techniques to assess cardiac function, preferably non-invasively, has
led to the development of several new diagnostic methods amongst which is cardiac
imaging. At the present time 3 different approaches are available, "cold spot" imaging - myocardial uptake or perfusion studies; "hot spot" imaging - for the localization of acutely ischemic areas of the myocardium; ventricular function - gated
blood pool imaging to provide regional and total ventricular function.

In this paper is reviewed the use of a short half-life (9.95 minute) positron emitter
Nitrogen-13 as labelled ammonia ($^{13}NH_4+$), a cold spot myocardial nuclide which can
be imaged using a standard gamma camera. More recently a novel form of positron
imaging has been developed to obtain back projection tomographic myocardial images,
anatomical localization of uptake defects and to quantitate the information collected.

MATERIALS AND METHODS

Nitrogen-13 labelled ammonia was produced in a small on-site medical cyclotron (C-S
15, Cyclotron Corporation), capable of accelerating protons to 15 MeV and deuterons
to 8 MeV. Originally $^{13}NH_4+$ was manufactured by the deuteron bombardment of Methane
as described by Tilbury et al. (1). Image quality, however, was shown to be incon-
sistent and occasionally very poor because of low contrast, since by this method
chemical purity of only 80% is possible. A new method of production was therefore
developed and introduced from 1973 onwards (2). Nitrogen-13 as nitrate was now produced by the proton bombardment of water and reduced by titanous hydroxide to ammonia
which was then recovered from the base by distillation within a few minutes. The
ammonia so produced has a radio-chemical purity of more than 99%; it contains less
than 15 - 20 ug of carrier ammonia per production run which takes about 8 minutes.

INSTRUMENTATION

In our earliest studies which began in 1971, imaging was performed using a Searle
Radiographics Pho-Gamma HP Scintillation Camera. Since our aim was to obtain scintigraphic information from patients without moving them from their ward to a central
laboratory area, mobility of the imaging apparatus was obtained by mounting the
scintillation camera on a mobile platform attached to a small electrical tractor. An
Ohio-Nuclear 150 Digital Data System was interfaced to the gamma camera and attached
as well to the electrical tractor, thus permitting the data to be acquired, stored
and processed in digital form at the patient's bedside.

Originally a standard 550 parallel-hole high-energy lead collimator was used. This
proved unsatisfactory because of septal thickness greater than resolution of the
system which resulted in the collimator hole pattern being conspicuously superimposed
on the image. Once this fault was recognized, a collimator of tungsten was specially
designed with the same hole size but with narrower septa. This increased the number
of holes, improved the collimator efficiency, reduced the hole pattern in the image

and has greatly improved overall image quality (3). More recently the tungsten collimator has been used in a rotating mode once more improving the overall quality of the images obtained. The improved quality of images obtained by these successive changes is shown in Figure 1.

A 20% pulse height-analyzer window centered around the 511 keV gamma energy peak from the positron annihilation of nitrogen-13 was used for imaging.

ANIMAL VALIDATION STUDIES

It is known that the pig has a coronary anatomy similar to that of man (4). A standard anterior infarct was created by ligating the left anterior descending coronary artery and in a second group of animals the first diagonal branch of the left anterior descending was ligated to produce anterolateral infarction. Technetium-99m labelled microspheres, 15 - 30 ug in diameter were injected directly into the left atrium and at the same time nitrogen-13 as ammonia was also injected. After sacrifices of the animals, 20 - 25 full thickness tissue samples through the infarct and the adjacent area of the myocardium were obtained, counted for nitrogen-13 activity and following decay of ^{13}N for ^{99m}Tc activity. The tissue sample counts of both nuclides were compared to injection standards and the percent of the injected dose of each agent per gram of tissue calculated.

Scintigraphic Anatomy

To determine scintigraphic anatomy the same animal model was used and a ^{99m}Tc point source placed at specific locations on the heart. The ^{99m}Tc images obtained were superimposed on ^{13}NH$_4$+ images following an intravenous injection of the nuclide thus providing an anatomically correct interpretation of nitrogen-13 ammonia myocardial images. On the basis of these animal studies myocardial scintigrams were divided into 4 segments: lateral, apical, inferior and septal. It was also possible to visually grade these images as (a) normal - homogenous and substantial (b) abnormal - localized uptake defect. When an uptake defect was present it could be further subdivided into a large segmental area (more than 50%) or small (less than 50%).

PATIENT STUDIES

Initially, 112 patients were investigated using intravenous ^{13}NH$_4$+. Myocardial scintigrams were obtained in the antero-posterior, left anterior oblique, and frequently right anterior oblique views, following the intravenous injection of 20 - 25 mCi carrier-free ^{13}NH$_4$+ at the patients' bedsides. The passage of the bolus of isotope through the heart was observed on a digital video display to insure correct patient positioning. Collection of images containing 1 million counts was begun immediately and continued until the count rate became too low, usually at about 30 minutes. Myocardial images obtained after pulmonary uptake had substantially cleared were used for interpretation once clear delineation of the lateral border of the heart was observed. Usually 2 - 4 million count images were available. Analog images were recorded on polaroid film and digitized scintillation data stored on magnetic tape in 10 second frames. No complications have resulted from the administration of intravenous nitrogen-13 as ammonia to more than 400 patients studied.

Following these initial studies, which were largely of patients with acute myocardial infarction immediately following admission to the coronary care unit, a study was done in an additional 50 patients to obtain sequential myocardial imaging throughout their hospital course following acute myocardial infarction. A separate group of patients with stable angina pectoris were also studied to determine the presence of scintigraphic uptake defects, first at rest and then during treadmill exercise testing. Many of these latter patients were re-studied both at rest and on exercise following coronary artery bypass graft surgery.

POSITRON IMAGING AND QUANTIFICATION OF UPTAKE DEFECTS

Whereas myocardial scintigraphy using the standard gamma camera approach as described above provides good visual representation of uptake defects, quantification of
such information poses formidable difficulties. One approach has been the development of a double camera system and of reconstructive 3-dimensional positron coincidence imaging, the data being presented as longitudinal or transverse tomographic
slices of the myocardium of any defined thickness and obtained simultaneously following a single injection of $^{13}NH_4$+ intravenously and the collection of count rates
over a 15 minute period.

Positron imaging is undertaken using a prototype apparatus constructed by Searle
Radiographics (5, 6, 7). Two large field conventional view scintillation cameras
are spaced 75 cms apart and mounted on a rotating gantry (Figure 2). The cameras
are operated in coincidence to detect annihilation radiation of the positron. The
following modifications have been made to insure adequate count rates, resolution
and sensitivity:-
The collimators were replaced by 10 inch diameter cyclindrical shields projecting
from the camera face and leaving the surfaces of the crystals exposed, thus excluding much of the ambient radiation originating in the body of the patient. Thin lead
absorbers (of about 1 mm in width) were placed over the crystal faces to exclude low
energy scattered radiation from the source. In addition, one inch thick crystals
replaced the usual half inch crystals of the gamma camera thus increasing its efficiency for detecting 511 keV radiations. Preamplifiers were modified to shorten the
integration times, and in addition DC coupled electronics were used to increase the
count rate capability.

A fast-slow coincidence system was used with a 10 ns gate to exclude all but coincident events from the slower pulse positioning and analyzing electronics.

The two cameras were operated using pulse-height windows of 20% centered on the 511
keV photopeak. Under operating conditions single counts of 300 - 400,000 for the
whole spectrum are tolerated. Some 1200 - 1500 counts per second of true coincident
events are obtained in the energy window when looking at the heart, and the random
rate is 5 - 10%. These desirable features are achieved with less than 1 mCi of
activity in the patient following an intravenous injection of $^{13}NH_4$+.

The data can be collected as uncorrected analog pictures in several planes whose
location and separation are variable. These images are largely used for monitoring
and positioning. The information is collected in parallel in list mode on tape and
subsequently processed by a computer to produce back projection images from which
the out of focus data is detected and corrected (8, 9). All images are normalized
to transmission images using a ^{68}Ge - ^{68}Ga sheet source to correct for the marked
radial variation of sensitivity, a result of solid angle variation and for varying
attenuation in the object under study.

RESULTS

Animal Experiments
Regional myocardial uptake of $^{13}NH_4$+ which was compared with the distribution of
^{99m}Tc-labelled microspheres showed an excellent correlation coefficient of 0.94 for
tissue uptake (measured as the percentage of injected dose per gram of tissue).
There was a low level of activity in the infarcted region, activity was high in the
apparently normal tissue and intermediate in the transitional zone of ischemia (Figure 3). It would appear therefore that the regional myocardial uptake of $^{13}NH_4$+ is
an appropriate reflection of the level of perfusion and similar to the tissue distribution of labelled microspheres (10, 11).

Patient Studies
Activity in the lungs cleared sufficiently to delineate the myocardial image in 3 -
36 minutes and was most rapid in non-smokers (mean 5.3 minutes) whereas it was slow-
est in smokers (mean 14.6 minutes). Significant uptake by the liver was also shown
and was maximal in the AP position but separation from the myocardium was obtained
in the LAO views (Figure 4). In no patient amongst many hundreds studied had the
information to be totally rejected because of lung or liver uptake.

Normal Controls
In normal individuals there is a homogenous myocardial image with a characteristic
"doughnut" configuration with a small area of reduced uptake between the septal and
lateral segments, corresponding to the regions of the aortic and mitral valves
(Figure 4). In addition, the apex of the left ventricle has reduced uptake since it
is thinner than other areas of the myocardium and is also subject to greater motion.

Disease States
In more than 96% of patients with acute myocardial infarction a characteristic
scintigraphic uptake defect was seen (Figure 5). Correspondence with the electrocardiographic localization of the infarct was good (12). Patients with infarction
at more than one site (recent or old) showed corresponding multiple perfusion defects
and in addition, other perfusion defects were frequently present even when the
electrocardiogram did not suggest additional lesions. For example, inferior perfusion defects were shown in the presence of acute anterior myocardial infarction.

Sequential imaging following acute myocardial infarction revealed rapid and dramatic
changes in the size of uptake defect which frequently was seen to vary day-to-day,
not infrequently heralding unsuspected clinical deterioration or confirming overall
clinical improvement in patients whose acute myocardial infarction was associated
with congestive cardiac failure (13). In addition, myocardial scintigraphy was
shown to be a sensitive index of the effects of various acute interventions used
therapeutically (14).

Patients with stable angina pectoris who were studied at rest and on exercise demonstrated uptake defects which worsened or which were brought out by exercise when the
myocardial scintigram was normal at rest. In those patients who went forward for
coronary artery bypass graft surgery, and in whom patency of the bypass grafts was
revealed by cardiac catheterization studies, post-operative myocardial scintigrams
showed great improvement in, or even absence of uptake defects which had been shown
pre-operatively.

Positron Imaging
Simultaneous longitudinal back projection tomographic images of the heart were obtained in the coronal plane in patients following acute myocardial infarction and
compared with routine gamma camera scintigrams. For both studies the nuclide used
was $^{13}NH_4+$ but because of the great sensitivity of the double-camera positron system
adequate counts were obtained using only 5 mCi injected intravenously and the study
was completed in 15 minutes. Much greater anatomical detail was obtained using the
new system and anatomical localization and extent of uptake defects were greatly
enhanced (Figure 6).

DISCUSSION

The development of pharmacological (15, 16), mechanical (17, 18), and surgical
techniques (19) to help support the ischemic myocardium adjacent to areas of infarction has been an important advance in patient management. A reliable non-invasive
method of assessing regional myocardial perfusion is needed. Myocardial imaging
using a short half-lived isotope such as nitrogen-13 labelled ammonia is a useful
approach since its uptake and distribution reflects tissue blood flow. To be sure

the need for an on-site cyclotron for its production does limit its use, but one can predict that as the advantages of accelerator produced nuclides become more apparent clinically, additional cyclotrons will become established at medical institutions (3).

Following an intravenous injection of $^{13}NH_4+$, blood disappearance is very rapid and 90% of the myocardial uptake occurs during its first pass. Only 15% of injected activity remains in the blood pool after 1 minute (20), thus the myocardial image can be visualized early without interference from blood pool background. Whereas organ distribution studies have shown that the liver is the principle site of uptake of $^{13}NH_4+$, containing approximately 15% of the injected dose, in man substantial uptake occurs as well in the brain, the heart, the lungs, the kidneys, the retina, and the bladder (20, 21). The uptake in the liver is slower than that in the myocardium reaching a peak approximately 10 minutes after injection and remaining constant throughout the procedure (20). Uptake by the lung is early and transient, except in chronic smokers; in them the explanation for delay in pulmonary clearing still remains obscure.

About 2 - 4% of the injected dose is taken up by the myocardium and in man it can be shown that this fraction remains constant for 30 minutes (20). The mechanism of uptake of ammonia by the myocardial cell has not yet been fully elucidated. Blood and disappearance kinetics suggest, however, that it probably differs from that of potassium and its analogs (20). NH_3 is freely permeable to cell membranes and at a physiological pH is predominantly in the ionized form (NH_4+), a relatively imperme-able cation (22). In other tissues, studies have demonstrated that NH_4+ may enter the cell by substituting for potassium and using the sodium-potassium ATP-ase dependent membrane system (23). Within the cell ammonia is metabolized via the glutamine synthetase pathway to glutamine which then enters the large body amino acid pool (23, 24, 25).

Whereas our animal studies have demonstrated that the myocardial uptake of $^{13}NH_4+$ parallels the distribution of microspheres in acute myocardial infarction, suggesting that the observed uptake defect represents areas of diminished or absent perfusion, it should be recognized that the defect is a resultant of at least 3 processes:- (1) perfusion, (2) transport into the region of interest, (3) metabolism by the myo-cardial cell. The defect seen on the scintigram may result from an abnormality of any one of these processes. No doubt the demonstration that in normals there is a homogenous myocardial uptake whereas in patients with obstructive coronary arterial disease localized uptake defects consistent with the abnormal regional perfusion occur, supports the belief that perfusion plays an important role in the consequent scintigram (26, 27).

Nitrogen-13 ammonia myocardial scintigraphy cannot distinguish between uptake defects, a result of myocardial infarction, or those due to other cardiac diseases. Thus ab-normal scintigrams are recorded frequently in patients with unstable angina, exacerb-ations of cardiac failure, acute cardiac rhythm disturbances, and stable angina pectoris with or without previous myocardial infarction. In the presence of old myo-cardial infarction a normal perfusion pattern suggests the development of adequate collateral circulation resulting in an improvement of regional perfusion to the damaged area. Certain patients with acute myocardial infarction who are imaged for some 20 - 30 minutes show a slower regional accumulation of nuclide activity occur-ring in certain regions of the myocardium, presumably under perfused or acutely ischemic segments. It is possible that the initial perfusion defect represents largely ischemic rather than necrotic myocardium which might allow sufficient tissue uptake of $^{13}NH_4+$ to occur, resulting eventually in a homogenous image being obtained.

Sequential studies on patients during the acute phase of myocardial infarction have shown that $^{13}NH_4+$ is a very suitable nuclide for frequent imaging studies in the same

patient. Since it has a very short half-life (9.95 minutes) there is only a modest
radiation dose to the patient. This has been calculated as 5 mRad/mCi to the whole
body and 25 mRad/mCi to the liver (20). A remarkable correlation between changes in
uptake defect and clinical status of the patient was seen (13). Myocardial scintigraphy using $^{13}NH_4+$ is helpful in assessing the prognosis of patients with acute
myocardial infarction and also in patients with unstable angina pectoris (12, 13,
14).

Since uptake defects vary dramatically with the clinical status of the patient, on
the one hand, and with therapeutic interventions on the other, it is unlikely that
standard myocardial scintigraphic information can be used as a measure of true size
of myocardial infarction.

The 3-dimensional shape and motion of the heart limits the diagnostic sensitivity
and specificity of 2-dimensional single projection imaging of $^{13}NH_4+$. While these
geometric problems can be overcome in part by imaging the heart in multiple projections, this increases the duration of the procedure. Accordingly, we began to investigate the use of tomographic myocardial scintigraphy in an attempt to resolve
the geometric limitations of standard gamma camera studies using the coincidence
detection of a positron emitter such as nitrogen-13 as ammonia. The fast-slow
coincidence system described permits operation with single count rates (whole spectrum) of 300 - 400,000 counts per second. Source scatter is excluded from the
detectors by specially designed graded absorbers resulting in a substantial increase
in sensitivity and the overall resolution is better than 10 mm. Images of tomographic back projections of planes whose location and separation is easily adjustable, parallel recording random events for use subsequently to correct the information being collected. The data is stored in a computer compatible record which was
processed originally using an IBM 370/168 computer but more recently using an Inter-
data 8/32 which offers the added advantage of on-line processing. Normalization to
a transmission image overcomes radial variation in sensitivity, corrects for variation of detector sensitivity and gives a first order correction for variation in
object attenuation. Longitudinal tomograms starting with single view back projections have been extensively investigated and more recently reconstructions from a
single view using the iterative method explored (19). To make the reconstructions
quantitative two problems remain to be solved:-
the first relates to better correction of attenuation of the transmission image in
tissue and the second to small angle scatter. It is hoped that additional work on
these problems will permit true quantification of the information to be obtained.

Positron imaging studies of the heart are also in progress at other institutions
(28). Furthermore intermediate cardiac metabolism may also be studied in man by
injecting fatty acids labelled with positron emitters such as carbon-11 (29), thus
opening an exciting new field of cardiac investigation at the cellular level in a
non-invasive manner.

CONCLUSION

The studies reported in this paper have shown that high quality, high count density
myocardial scintigrams can be obtained in man using intravenous nitrogen-13 ammonia
and a mobile scintillation camera. This method is reliable and safe even in very
ill patients for the detection of myocardial uptake defects. It is especially useful when serial myocardial imaging at short intervals is needed. The motion and 3-
dimensional geometry of the heart limit the accuracy of conventional imaging techniques in defining uptake defects anatomically, but positron imaging using a double
gamma camera system suitably modified and the development of computer algorithms
provides back projection longitudinal tomograms in the coronal plane which largely
overcome the geometric and technological problems of routine gamma camera myocardial
scintigraphy. The new method furthermore, is capable of quantifying the information
obtained and of providing an accurate anatomical assessment of position and extent
of myocardial uptake defects.

REFERENCES

(1) Tilbury, R.S., Dahl, J.R., Monahan, W.G. and Laughlin, J.S. (1971): Radiochem. Radioanal. Letters, 8, 317.

(2) Lathrop, K.A., Harper, P.V., Rich, B.H., Dinwoodie, R., Krizek, H., Lembares, N. and Gloria, I. (1973): In: Radiopharmaceuticals and Labelled Compounds, Vienna, International Atomic Energy Agency, 1973. pp. 471-481, Vol. I.

(3) Harper, P.V., Schwartz, J., Beck, R.N., Lathrop, K.A., Lembares, N., Krizek, H., Gloria, I., Dinwoodie, R., McLaughlin, A., Stark, V.J., Bekerman, C., Hoffer, P.B., Gottschalk, A., Resnekov, L., Al-Sadir, J., Mayorga, A. and Brooks, H.L. (1973): Radiology, 108, 613.

(4) Bertho, E. and Gagnon, G. (1964): Dis. Chest, 46, 251.

(5) Muehllehner, G. (1975): J. Nucl. Med., 16, 653.

(6) Muehllehner, G., Buchin, M.P. and Dudek, J.H. (1976): IEEE Transactions NS, 23, 528.

(7) Muehllehner, G., Atkins, F., Harper, P. et al. (1976): Proc. IAEA Symposium, Los Angeles, October, 1976. (In press).

(8) Atkins, F.B., Oppenheim, B.E. and Harper, P.V. (1976): Proc. 4th Int. Congr. on Medical Physics, Ottawa, 1976.

(9) Huang, T.S., Barker, D.A. and Berger, S.P. (1975): Appl. Optics, 14, 1165.

(10) Domenech, R.J., Hoffman, J.I.E., Noble, M.I.M., Saunders, K.B., Henson, J.R. and Subijanto, S. (1969): Circ. Res., 25, 581.

(11) Uttey, J., Carlson, E.L., Hoffman, J.I.E., Martinez, H.M. and Buckberg, G.D. (1974): Circ. Res., 34, 391.

(12) Walsh, W.F., Harper, P.V., Resnekov, L. and Fill, H. (1976): Circulation, 54, 266.

(13) Karunaratne, H., Walsh, W., Fill, H., Harper, P. and Resnekov, L. (1976): Circulation, 54, Suppl. 2:II, 76.

(14) Walsh, W., Harper, P., Resnekov, L. and Fill, H. (1976): Clin. Res., 24, 245A.

(15) Miller, R.R., Vismara, L.A., Zelis, R., Amsterdam, E.A. and Mason, D.T. (1975): Circulation, 51, 328.

(16) Willerson, J.T., Curry, G.C., Atkins, J.M., Parkey, R. and Horwitz, L.D. (1975): Circulation, 51, 1095.

(17) Gold, H.K., Leinbach, R.C., Sanders, C.A., Buckley, M.J., Mundth, E.D. and Austen, W.G. (1973): Circulation, 47, 1197.

(18) Leinbach, R.C., Gold, H.K., Buckley, M.J., Austen, W.G. and Sanders, C.A. (1973): Circulation, 48, Suppl. 4:IV, 100.

(19) Cooley, D.A., Dawson, J.T., Hallman, G.L., Sandiford, F.M., Wukasch, D.C., Garcia, E. and Hall, R.J. (1973): Ann. Thorac. Surg., 16, 380.

(20) Harper, P.V., Lathrop, K.A., Krizek, H., Lembares, N., Stark, V. and Hoffer, P.B. (1972): J. Nucl. Med., 13, 278.

(21) Monahan, W.G., Tilbury, R.S. and Laughlin, J.S. (1972): J. Nucl. Med., 13, 274.

(22) Davidson, S. and Sonnenblick, E.H. (1975): Cardiovasc. Res., 9, 295.

(23) Post, R.L. and Jolly, P.C. (1957): Biochim. Biophys. Acta, 25, 118.

(24) Kato, T. (1968): Jap. Circ. J., 32, 1401.

(25) Watanabe, T. (1968): Jap. Circ. J., 32, 1811.

(26) Jansen, C., Grames, G.M. and Judkins, M.P. (1974): In: Cardiovascular Nuclear Medicine. Eds. Strauss, H.W., Pitt, B. and James, E.A. New York, CV Mosby Company, pp. 211.

(27) Cannon, P.J., Schmidt, D.H., Weiss, M.B., Fowler, D.L., Sciacca, R.R., Kent, E. and Casarella, W.J. (1975): J. Clin. Invest., 56, 1442.

(28) Hoffman, E.J., Phelps, M. and Mullani, N. (1976): J. Nucl. Med., 17, 493.

(29) Ter-Pogossian, M.M., Hoffman, E.J., Weiss, E.S., Coleman, R.E., Phelps, M.E., Welch, M.J. and Sobel, B.E. (1975): In: Proceedings of the Conference on Cardiovascular Imaging and Image Processing Theory and Practice. Eds. Harrison, D.C., Sandler, H. and Miller, H.A. Palos Verdes Estates. Society of Photo-optical Instrumentation Engineers, 1975, p. 277, Vol. 72.

Dr. Dennis Krikler asked whether Dr. Resnekov had used scintigraphy for the assessment of response to pharmacological agents in patients with cardiac infarction: Dr. Resnekov thought that this would be valuable for assessing changes in jeopardised myocardium. He agreed with Professor Desmond Julian and Dr. Lawson McDonald that scintigraphy could be combined with coronary arteriography in selection of patients for surgery. Dr. Robert Bruce underlined the value of scintigraphy in showing the redistribution of blood from the viscera (e.g. liver) to the heart, which occurs during myocardial infarction and also during exercise; Dr. Resnekov stressed that this was a sensitive method of showing such changes.

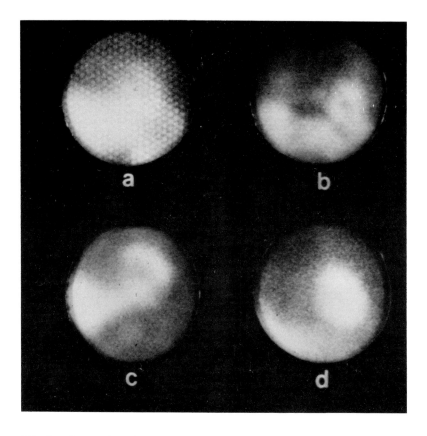

FIG. 1   Improved quality of myocardial scintigrams.
A.   Poor quality scintigram. $^{13}NH_4^+$ was produced by deuteron bombardment of methane and is only 80% pure. Pattern of the lead collimator superimposed on image.
B.   A specially designed tungsten collimator is substituted but $^{13}NH_4^+$ is still only 80% pure.
C.   Tungsten collimator and injecting 99% pure $^{13}NH_4^+$ produced by proton bombardment of water.
D.   Rotating tungsten collimator and using 99% pure $^{13}NH_4^+$ has resulted in myocardial scintigrams of diagnostic quality.

146

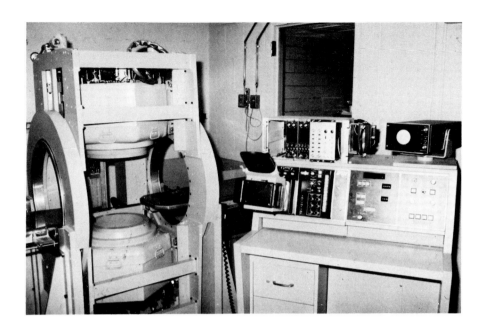

FIG. 2   Prototype double-camera assembly mounted on a rotating gantry and special electronics for positron imaging of the heart following an intravenous injection of $^{13}NH_4^+$.

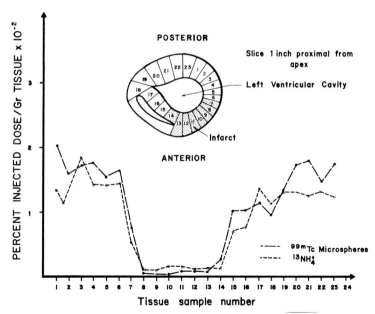

FIG. 3   Comparison of regional uptake of $^{13}NH_4^+$ with the distribution of ^{99m}Tc-labelled microspheres across created myocardial infarction in the pig. The percentage injected dose/gram of tissue for both agents is plotted for the tissue samples arranged in anatomical continuity.   (Reproduced by permission (12)).

147

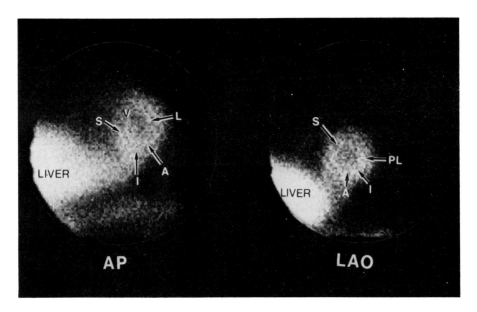

FIG. 4   Normal myocardial scintigram in the antero-posterior (AP) and left anterior
oblique (LAO) projections following an intravenous injection of $^{13}NH_4^+$.
S = septum. L = lateral. A = apex. I = inferior. PL = postero-lateral.
V = region of aortic and mitral valves. (Reproduced by permission (12)).

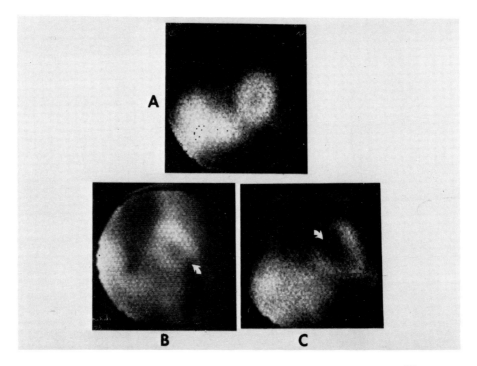

FIG. 5   Myocardial scintigraphy following an intravenous injection of $^{13}NH_4^+$.
A - Normal
B - Inferior myocardial infarct, arrowed.
C - Anteroseptal myocardial infarct, arrowed.

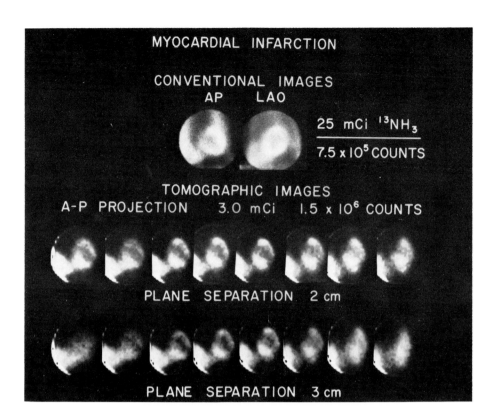

FIG. 6   Conventional imaging above and immediately consecutive reconstructed back
          projection longitudinal tomography positron images in the coronal plane
          below, in a patient with old antero-septal and recent postero-lateral
          myocardial infarction.

          Conventional imaging in the AP view shows rather subtle uptake defects in
          the septum and apex with the postero-lateral defect clearly shown in the
          LAO view in which the subtle defect of the apex is also seen.

          Greatly improved delineation is seen in the reconstructed tomographic posi-
          tron images particularly with a plane separation of 2 cms. A large uptake
          defect extends from the septum across the anterior wall to the apex where
          a large defect is obvious. The postero-lateral defect can be seen in the
          deeper cuts (right).

          Note that the tomographic images were obtained simultaneously following an
          injection of only 3 mCi of the nuclide.

CORONARY ARTERIOGRAPHY

P.S. Robinson and John Coltart

(This Section was prepared by the authors, at short notice, as the manuscript of
Melvin Judkins was not available. Incorporated are notes made by P.S.R. on
Dr. Judkins' communications)

Selective coronary arteriography is the standard technique whereby the presence of
coronary arterial disease is established, by which coronary arterial anatomy is
determined and against which non-invasive techniques for the detection of coronary
arterial disease are judged. Improvement in catheters and catheterisation techniques
have rendered the procedure safe, although not entirely free of risk, and improvement
in x-ray equipment, particularly the image intensifier, have enabled the rapid
production of high resolution images on 35 mm. cine-film and on 70 mm. or 100 mm.
spot films. The purpose of this presentation is to review these improvements and to
consider the indications and problems of coronary arteriography in the diagnosis and
management of overt and latent coronary arterial disease.

Recent Improvements

The earlier image intensifiers used zinc cadmium sulphide as the input phosphor.
Using these image intensifiers with the x-ray generators then available the diagnostic quality of cine-films was poor, particularly with regard to small vessel anatomy
and high-resolution images could only be obtained using large films and long
exposures. The new generation of image intensifiers employ caesium iodide as the
input phosphor. The auxillary electrodes in the electron-optical path have been
refined and exposure setting is now automatic. X-ray generators produce brief pulses
of x-rays and using exposure times of less than 8 milliseconds blurring due to movement is reduced to a minimum. With these improvements and using medium speed fine
grain films instead of high speed coarse grain films previously employed, it is
possible to produce high resolution 35 mm. cine-films, and 70 mm. or 100 mm. spot
films without loss of diagnostic information compared to the images previously
obtained by large film techniques (1). A further factor likely to improve the diagnostic yield of coronary arteriography is the mounting of the x-ray tube and image
intensifier on a rotating U-arm. This simplifies positioning for oblique projections
and allows cranio-caudal angulation to examine the left main coronary artery, the
proximal left anterior descending coronary artery and its diagonal and septal branches. The final place of these views in routine coronary arteriography has yet to be
determined but in a study of 2,500 cases Bruschke found significantly improved diagnostic information in 4% using cranio-caudal views routinely (2). Preshaped thermo-
plastic catheters have greatly simplified selective intubation of the coronary ostia
and continuous pressure monitoring during intubation and before and after contrast
injection has improved the safety of the procedure. With experience mortality and
complication rates are low regardless of whether the brachial or femoral route is
employed and there is evidence that the systemic administration of heparin has reduced the incidence of thrombo-embolic complications.

Clinical Manifestations of Coronary Arterial Disease

Before considering the indications for coronary arteriography, it will be useful to outline the clinical manifestations of coronary arterial disease, the factors influencing prognosis, the stages in investigation and the non-invasive tests currently employed in the investigation of coronary arterial disease. The clinical manifestations of coronary arterial disease are outlined in Table 1.

TABLE 1

Clinical Manifestations of Coronary Arterial Disease

Chronic stable angina pectoris

Unstable angina pectoris

Ventricular arrhythmias

Acute myocardial infarction

The complications of myocardial infarction

        Left ventricular aneurysm

        Ventricular septal defect

        Papillary muscle dysfunction

        Ventricular arrhythmias

Sudden death

Latent coronary arterial disease

        With evidence of myocardial ischaemia

        With no detectable abnormality

The minimal disease found in angina pectoris is 80% stenosis of a single coronary artery and angina commonly implies severe disease of at least two coronary arteries. The other common presentation of coronary artery disease is acute myocardial infarction or more rarely the complications of infarction: left ventricular aneurysm, ventricular septal defect, papillary muscle dysfunction or ventricular arrhythmias. The Framingham Study showed that only 23% of patients suffering myocardial infarction had a preceding history of angina pectoris while in the majority myocardial infarction was the first manifestation of coronary arterial disease. Patients resuscitated following sudden cardiac death (generally ventricular fibrillation) frequently do not subsequently develop evidence of acute myocardial infarction. The risk of recurrent ventricular fibrillation in these patients over the following months and years is high and they almost invariably have severe coronary arterial disease often with anatomy suitable for coronary arterial surgery (3, 4, 5). Overt manifestation of coronary arterial disease thus generally implies severe coronary arterial disease. Early detection of coronary arterial disease requires detection prior to irreversible myocardial damage and generally prior to the onset of symptoms - latent coronary arterial disease. In some asymptomatic patients there is detectable evidence of myocardial ischaemia either at rest - ventricular arrhythmias, or during exercise stress - ST segment changes or arrhythmias on electrocardiography or haemodynamic abnormalities. Myocardial perfusion imaging occasionally reveals evidence of myocardial ischaemia in the absence of the abnormalities outlined above. Occasionally patients with latent coronary arterial disease with no detectable physiological abnormalities are found to have disease when coronary arteriography is undertaken in 'high risk' patients with either a hyperlipidaemia or a family history of severe coronary arterial disease.

The prognosis of the patient with coronary arterial disease is predominantly determined by two factors which may be determined at coronary arteriography. These are
1) the extent of coronary arterial disease and 2) left ventricular function. In
1973 Bruschke and his associates reviewed the Cleveland Clinic experience of 590
consecutive non-surgical cases of angiographically documented coronary arterial
disease followed for at least 5 years. Five year mortality is outlined in Table 2
and demonstrates the influence of the extent of coronary arterial disease and the
appearance of the left ventricle on cine-angiography. Their figures showed that the
clinical presentation and the presence of risk factors had little influence on
survival (6, 7). Improvements in medical treatment since this study was completed
have reduced the mortality slightly but overall trends remain unchanged.

Therapeutic decision-making, therefore, depends on establishing the presence of
coronary arterial disease and assessing the extent and severity of the disease and
the state of the left ventricle.

TABLE 2

5 Year Mortality in Angiographically Documented Coronary

Arterial Disease (Bruschke 1973)

		5 year mortality
1.	Number of vessels with ⟩ 50% stenosis:	
	Isolated single vessel disease	7%
	Single vessel disease with other minor disease	23%
	Double vessel disease	38%
	Triple vessel disease	54%
	Left main coronary arterial disease	57%
2.	Appearance of the left ventricle on cine-angiography:	
	Normal	25%
	Localised scar	31%
	Aneurysm	46%
	Diffuse scar	69%

The sequence for investigation is outlined in Table 3.

TABLE 3

Therapeutic Decision Making - Investigation Sequence

History

Clinical examination

Assessment of risk factors

Resting electrocardiogram

Chest x-ray

Stress testing - electrocardiography

               - myocardial imaging

Coronary arteriography and evaluation of collaterals

Left ventricular cine-angiography and assessment of
   left ventricular function

The extent to which this sequence is followed depends on the clinical situation and
this will be discussed in detail with the indications for coronary arteriography.
Non-invasive studies are widely employed in the investigation of coronary arterial
disease - particularly exercise stress testing with electrocardiographic monitoring.
The electrocardiographic manifestations of ischaemia have been discussed in a
previous contribution to this symposium (Robinson and Coltart). The incidence of
false negative investigations has been stressed and depending on the prevalence of
coronary arterial disease in the population under consideration there may be a
substantial number of false positive results. Myocardial perfusion imaging particularly using thallium 201 improves the sensitivity of exercise testing but a number
of false negative investigations persist. The incidence of false positive results
should markedly diminish but the final place of myocardial imaging has yet to be
determined. Coronary arteriography remains the objective standard for the diagnosis
of coronary arterial disease.

Indications for coronary arteriography

The indications for coronary arteriography are listed in Table 4 and have been considered in detail in a recent report from the ad hoc Committee on the Indications for
Coronary Arteriography (8). Careful distinction is made between the research needs
of specialised centres and the requirements for informed management of the patient
with coronary arterial disease in the clinical setting. This report also stresses
the acceptable risks and quality-control required of a unit undertaking this investigation. The incidence of complications should be carefully monitored.

The use of coronary arteriography to elucidate chest pain of uncertain origin should
be considered if, despite careful study including stress testing, there remains a
definite suspicion of coronary arterial disease and if a firm diagnosis is considered
essential for future management. Of course, the finding of coronary arterial disease
does not prove a causal relationship with the symptoms. In certain essential
occupations related to public safety such as air-line pilots the information obtained
from coronary arteriography may be critical for future management.

154

TABLE 4

The Indications for Coronary Arteriography

A. Specialised research needs

B. Patient management

Elective:	Chest pain of uncertain origin	
	Stable angina pectoris	
	Ventricular arrhythmias	
	Valvar or congenital heart disease	
Acute phase:	Unstable angina pectoris	
	Sudden cardiac arrest	
	Acute myocardial infarction	
	Complications of infarction	
		left ventricular failure
		papillary muscle dysfunction
		ventricular septal defect
		left ventricular aneurysm

Following myocardial infarction

Following aorto-coronary bypass surgery

Latent coronary arterial disease

Prolongation of life by coronary surgery in the absence of left main coronary arterial disease has not been clearly established. However, if it were proved that longevity in double or triple vessel disease with good left ventricular function was improved following surgery then the indications for coronary arteriography might be considerably broadened. At present in the situation of chronic stable angina pectoris, arteriography should be undertaken for severe angina refractory to medical treatment and compromising the desired quality of life, since this group of patients should be considered for surgery for relief of pain. Coronary arteriography for evaluation of prognosis alone is probably unjustified since medical management short of surgery should not be different. Refractory ventricular arrhythmias have, on occasion, been successfully treated by revascularising surgery with or without aneurysmectomy, and warrant investigation. The incidence of coronary arterial disease in valvar heart disease (particularly aortic valvar disease) is sufficiently high to justify arteriography in the routine preoperative evaluation of such patients - certainly over the age of 40.

In the acute phase of coronary arterial disease coronary arteriography may be considered in certain defined situations. In unstable angina pectoris there is, as yet, no conclusive evidence of prolongation of life or prevention of infarction by early surgery and there appear to be no disadvantages to aggressive medical management initially with coronary arteriography if pain persists or electively at 3 months. New onset angina pectoris, per se, is not an indication for coronary arteriography unless the situation is unstable or the symptoms are severe and refractory to medical treatment. Resuscitation following sudden cardiac arrest represents a 'high risk' situation and investigation should be undertaken. Following acute myocardial infarction revascularising surgery carries a high mortality and evidence of salvage of compromised myocardium is inconclusive. Investigation by coronary arteriography should be reserved for life threatening complications where high risk surgical intervention may be justified. In the convalescent phase of myocardial infarction some authorities recommend routine investigation to determine prognosis and future management about 3 months after infarction. The diagnosis is not in doubt and the results of surgery in prolonging life and preventing infarction are uncertain so that at present investigation should probably be restricted to those with persistent symptoms. Following aorto-coronary bypass surgery repeat coronary arteriography is not essential. Graft patency rates and the relationship between symptomatic and functional results and successful revascularisation are sufficiently well established to enable routine post-operative assessment by exercise testing, electrocardiography and myocardial imaging. In the presence of continuing or recurrent symptoms reinvestigation is justified.

Latent coronary arterial disease presents another situation in which the decision to undertake coronary arteriography is controversial. In a research setting it is necessary to establish screening procedures such as myocardial perfusion imaging; the significance of changes on the exercise electrocardiogram are well established. Until surgery can be shown to confer definite benefit in terms of prolongation of life and prevention of infarction then coronary arteriography should not be considered routine in the asymptomatic patient detected by screening procedures or in the high risk patient with hyperlipidaemia or a strong family history of coronary arterial disease.

Left main stem coronary arterial disease represents a special situation in which there is little doubt that surgery improves survival. However, the patient with left main stem coronary arterial disease generally has severe and often unstable angina frequently with rest pain, and exercise testing usually shows considerable restriction of exercise capacity with gross ST segment changes at low work loads and failure of the pressor response to exercise. These patients would be detected and investigated on the criteria discussed above. The yield of left main stem disease in asymptomatic patients, following uncomplicated acute infarction and in all patients with new onset of angina would undoubtedly be low and probably would not justify the extensive investigation required to detect it. In addition left main coronary arterial disease has not been identified as a particular risk factor in sudden cardiac death. In all patients with coronary arterial disease documented at coronary arteriography the incidence of left main stem coronary arterial disease is approximately 3% with isolated left main stem coronary arterial disease in 0.1 to 0.5% (6, 9).

Complications of Coronary Arteriography

The risks of coronary arteriography include death, myocardial infarction, coronary arterial dissection or embolism, ventricular arrhythmias, thrombosis or false aneurysm formation at the arterial entry site, and cerebral embolism. It should be stressed that with good technique the risks are proportional to the condition of the patient at the time of the examination. Also as Judkins states "an unheralded complication of coronary arteriography frequently overlooked but equal in importance to the most severe, is an incomplete or non-diagnostic study" - this may lead to inappropriate medical or surgical treatment or to the risks of a repeat investigation. In 1973 Adams reviewed the risks of coronary arteriography from published studies and compared the femoral and brachial approaches (10). This was prior to the use of systemic heparinisation and certainly the complication rates from the femoral approach would not be acceptable today particularly for the wide range of indications discussed above. Table 5 outlines the results compiled by Adams and also documents the complications from the laboratories of Judkins and of Bourassa recently presented (11, 12). Both the latter investigators employ the femoral approach using pre-shaped catheters. The routine use of heparin has been shown by Judkins to reduce thromboembolism and he has also demonstrated, by the use of "pull-out" angiograms of the femoral artery, a reduced incidence of local femoral thrombus formation around the catheter entry site. Care with catheter tip manipulation around the coronary ostia and continuous pressure monitoring throughout the catheter are important aids to a low risk procedure.

TABLE 5

	n	Death	Myocardial Infarction	Arterial Thrombosis	Cerebral Embolism
Adams (1973)					
Brachial	22142	0.13%	0.22%	1.67%	0.03%
Femoral	22780	0.78%	1.01%	1.19%	0.43%
Bourassa (1975)					
no heparin	5251	0.23%	0.09%	0.68%	0.13%
Judkins (1975)					
no heparin	7000	0.07%	0.12%	0.3%	0.13%
heparin	880	-	-	0.11%	-

Chest Pain with Normal Coronary Arteries

Of interest has been the emergence of a group of patients with chest pain suggestive of coronary arterial disease but with normal vessels at coronary arteriography; these are outlined in Table 6.

TABLE 6

Chest Pain with Normal Coronary Arteries

Coronary embolism

Recanalised coronary arterial thrombosis

Coronary arterial spasm

Syndrome X

Mitral leaflet prolapse

Anomalous origin of the left coronary artery

Myocardial 'bridging'

An occasional patient is seen who at coronary arteriography for investigation of chest pain is demonstrated to have intra-arterial defects which are not present at subsequent investigations. This may represent transient arterial thrombus formation with subsequent thrombolysis. These patients are usually young and not infrequently are women taking oral contraceptives. Thrombosis with recanalisation may explain a group of similar patients who sustain myocardial infarction but are subsequently found to have normal coronary arteries. Coronary arterial spasm is frequently seen at coronary arteriography and appears to be of two types. "Non-ischaemic" spasm is probably provoked by the catheter tip or contrast injection and there are no associated symptoms or haemodynamic changes. "Ischaemic" spasm is accompanied by chest pain, ST segment elevation and reduction in left ventricular function, and appears to be the basis of variant or Prinzmetal angina. The spasm may be a response to catecholamines and is abolished by glyceryl trinitrate. Syndrome X is a less well defined entity consisting of anginal-type chest pain, normal coronary arteries and "ischaemic" ST segment depression during atrial pacing - left ventricular function improves, with reduction of left ventricular end-diastolic pressure, on pacing, in contradistinction to the situation with obstructive coronary arterial disease. This probably represents a cardiomyopathy. Mitral leaflet prolapse is a common condition in young women in which systolic clicks are associated with chest pain, particularly at rest and sometimes severe, arrhythmias, "ischaemic" ST segment depression on pacing, abnormal lactate metabolism and either hypokinesia or hyperkinesia on left ventricular cine-angiography. This may also represent a cardiomyopathy. Exertional chest pain has rarely been described with anomalous origin of the left coronary artery from the right sinus of Valsalva. The artery courses between aorta and pulmonary artery and may be compressed as arterial pressures rise with exertion. This anomaly has been recorded as a rare cause of sudden death (13). An intra-myocardial segment of an epicardial artery is occasionally described and may similarly be responsible for chest pain.

Anomalies of Coronary Arterial Anatomy

The major importance of congenital anomalies in the origin of the coronary arteries lies in the confusion which may arise at coronary arteriography if the ostia are not cannulated, particularly in patients undergoing evaluation for coronary arterial surgery. In a series of 4250 patients undergoing coronary arteriography anomalous origin of one or more coronary arteries was described in 55 (1.3%) (14). The commonest anomaly was origin of the circumflex coronary artery from the right sinus of Valsalva.

REFERENCES

(1) Judkins, M.P. and Gander, M.P. (1973): Circulation, 47, IV, 89.
(2) Bruschke, A.V.G. and Ludwig, J.W. (1975): Cranio-caudal projections in coronary arteriography. Coronary arteriography and angina pectoris. Symposium of the European Society of Cardiology, 22. Ed. P.R. Lichtlen, Georg Thieme, Stuttgart.
(3) Myerburg, R.J., Ghahramani, A., Mallon, S.M., Castellanos, A. and Kaiser, G. (1975): Circulation, 52, Suppl. III, 219.
(4) Cobb, L.A., Baum, R.S., Alvarez, H. and Schaffe, W.A. (1975): Circulation, 52, Suppl. III, 223.
(5) Weaver, W.D., Lorch, G.S., Alvarez, H.A. and Cobb, L.A. (1976): Circulation, 54, 895.
(6) Bruschke, A.V.G., Proudfit, W.L. and Sones, L.M. (1973): Circulation, 47, 1147.
(7) Bruschke, A.V.G., Proudfit, W.L. and Sones, L.M. (1973): Circulation, 47, 1154.
(8) Bristow, J.D., Burchell, H.B., Campbell, R.W., Ebert, P.A., Hall, R.J., Leonard, J.J. and Reeves, T.J. (1977): Circulation, 55, 969A.
(9) Takaro, T., Hultgren, H.N., Lipton, M.J. and Detre, K.M. (1976): Circulation, 54, Suppl. III, 107.
(10) Adams, D.F., Fraser, D.B. and Abrams, H.L. (1973): Circulation, 48, 609.
(11) Gander, M.P. and Judkins, M.P. (1975): Advances in coronary arteriography using the Judkins technique. Coronary arteriography and angina pectoris. Symposium of the European Society of Cardiology, 26. Ed. P.R. Lichtlen, Georg Thieme, Stuttgart.
(12) Bourassa, M.G. and Lésperance, J. (1975): New advances with the Bourassa technique of coronary arteriography. Coronary arteriography and angina

pectoris. <u>Symposium of the European Society of Cardiology, 31</u>. Ed. P.R.
Lichtlen, Georg Thieme, Stuttgart.

(13) Cheitlin, M.D., de Castro, C.M. and McAllister, H.A. (1974): <u>Circulation</u>, 50,
780.

(14) Engel, H.J. and Page, H.L. (1975): Angiographic demonstration of variations
in coronary anatomy. Coronary arteriography and angina pectoris. <u>Symposium
of the European Society of Cardiology, 44</u>. Ed. P.R. Lichtlen, Georg Thieme,
Stuttgart.

QUESTIONS

<u>Dr. Oscar Magidson</u> asked about the importance of myocardial "bridges" as obstruct-
ive lesions; <u>Dr. Judkins</u> agreed that they occurred, albeit rarely, considering them
of particular importance if they were thick or long.

CORONARY VASOSPASM AS A CAUSE OF ANGINA PECTORIS

Attilio Maseri

Laboratory of the National Council for Research, Pisa

For a long time coronary spasm was considered to be one of the causes of angina pectoris on clinical grounds (1, 2, 3). This hypothesis was completely discarded following the observation that significant coronary atherosclerotic obstructions were
found at necroscopy in nearly all anginal patients (4). On the basis of this observation the notion arose that angina pectoris was "secondary" to an increase of myocardial metabolic demand which exceeded the possibility of coronary blood supply,
limited by the presence of coronary atherosclerotic obstructions. Thus prominent
cardiology text books (5) taught: "The occurrence of the pain or pressure with effort is an essential element of the syndrome .... it may occur at rest, but if it
does not also occur with effort .... the diagnosis of angina pectoris may be
questioned".

This unilateral concept has so far profoundly conditioned both the interpretation of
the symptomatology of the patients and the consequent medical and surgical therapy
of angina pectoris.

The traditional concept that angina ensues whenever oxygen supply is short of myocardial metabolic demand because of the presence of coronary artery stenosis, was challenged by the finding that about 10% of the patients thought to have unmistakable
angina, have normal coronary arteriograms (6, 7, 8, 9) and by the studies of Guazzi
et al. (10) indicating that in patients with "variant" angina, the attacks were not
preceded by any increase of the hemodynamic parameters controlling myocardial oxygen
consumption. Thus in these patients, angina cannot be considered "secondary" to an
increased myocardial demand, and a "primary" origin should be postulated (11).

Among the possible causes of "primary" angina (vasospasm, platelet aggregation, myocardial metabolic alterations) vasospasm deserves particular attention because it
has been observed during attacks of "variant" angina in a number of isolated occasi-
ons at coronary arteriography, more by chance than by design (12, 13, 14, 15).

With the purpose of elucidating the pathogenic mechanism of unstable angina (16) at
rest, in particular of the "crescendo" type (17, 18), in 1973 we undertook a series
of multidisciplinary, coordinated studies most of which have just been published.
We performed: (1) hemodynamic monitoring, in order to investigate whether or not
the anginal attacks were preceded by an increase of myocardial demand (19, 20, 21,
22); (2) radioisotopic myocardial perfusion studies during the attack, in order to
evidence the possible occurrence of localized reduction of perfusion (23, 24); (3)
coronary angiography during the attack in order to document the possible occurrence
of vasospasm and its location (21, 22, 23, 24, 25, 26). Hemodynamic monitoring proved that these patients had "primary" angina, and showed that the sequence of the
events during each attack was remarkably similar to that observed following abrupt
experimental coronary occlusion. Radioisotopic studies confirmed that during the
attack a massive reduction of myocardial perfusion was present, with a transmural
distribution in anginal attacks characterized by S-T segment elevation and with a
subendocardial distribution in those characterized by S-T segment depression. Angiographic studies during the attack showed a diffuse occlusive spasm of a large vess-

el in patients with transmural ischemia and spasm of minor branches, or diffuse, but incomplete spasm, or presence of collaterals, in those with subendocardial ischemia. In this presentation we wish to summarize the results of these studies and to discuss the implications of the demonstration of coronary spasm in the diagnostic evaluation and on the management of these patients without entering the discussion on the pathogenesis of spasm.

Hemodynamic Monitoring

We have performed continuous hemodynamic monitoring during 10-14 hours in 22 patients referred to our C.C.U. because of "crescendo" angina. A combination of the following parameters was monitored: 1 to 4 ECG leads (in all); left ventricular pressure (18 pts) or aortic and pulmonary artery pressure (4 pts), right ventricular pressure (13 pts), pulmonary artery mixed venous oxygen saturation (8 pts), coronary sinus oxygen saturation (3 pts). A total of 337 episodes of acute transient myocardial ischemia, recorded on a 14 Track magnetic tape recorder (Analog 14 Philips) were of sufficiently good technical quality. They could be played back on photographic paper and different speeds for inspective or manual analysis and converted into digital form for computer analysis (21, 22).

In 4 patients no episodes were observed during the monitoring period; we observed only episodes of S-T segment elevation in 13 patients, only of S-T segment depression in 3 and alternating episodes of S-T elevation and depression in the same leads in 2 patients.

The attacks were never preceded by consistent changes of heart rate or blood pressure (Figure 1A, 1B) the S-T segment changes were generally preceded by a drop of coronary sinus oxygen saturation (Figure 2) a sharp drop of relaxation peak dp/dt, of contraction peak dp/dt, of systolic pressure and by an increase of end-diastolic pressure, as observed in the dog during experimental coronary occlusion (27, 28, 29) the changes were usually abrupt in the episodes of S-T segment elevation and gradual in those of S-T segment depression although in both similar levels of left ventricular end-diastolic pressure (up to 50 mm Hg) could be observed. Pain was always a late phenomenon and was absent in an appreciable number of episodes of acute, transient ischemia (Figure 3). These findings confirm and extend those of Guazzi (10, 30) but are in disagreement with other reports which, erroneously, considered pain as the onset of the ischemic attack and, observing increased values of heart rate and systolic blood pressure at this time, considered these changes as responsible for the attack (31, 32).

Myocardial Scintigraphy

We were able to perform myocardial scintigraphy with thallium-201 in 37 patients during attacks of angina at rest; 23 presented with S-T segment elevation, 2 with pseudonormalization of basally inverted "T" waves; 12 with S-T segment depression. The attack occurred spontaneously in 11 patients and was induced by intravenous injection of ergonovine maleate 0.05 to 0.20 mg in 26.

Scintigrams were obtained on a Jumbo Toshiba gamma camera on a 35 x 35 cm film, in multiple projections immediately after the injection (5 to 20 min) and about 3 hours later, scintigraphy was repeated at a week's distance following Thallium-201 in the absence of symptoms, with the same modalities.

In all patients with S-T elevation or with pseudonormalization of "T" waves a massive transmural deficit of perfusion was observed (Figure 4). The alterations were generally less obvious in patients with S-T segment depression, who showed a diffuse reduction of perfusion involving predominantly one wall in 6 patients, the subendocardial portion of one wall in 2 patients (Figure 5) and the whole heart in 3 patients; in the last patient no obvious defects of perfusion were apparent probably because myocardial ischemia was relieved too early after the injection of the radionuclide (23, 24, 33).

These studies document that the anginal attacks at rest are accompanied by appreciable reduction of myocardial perfusion which appear to be transmural during S-T segment elevation or pseudonormalization of "T" waves and subendocardial during S-T segment depression. Thus the similarity of the hemodynamic findings during anginal attacks with those observed during experimental coronary occlusion, finds further support in the objective demonstration of a reduced regional myocardial perfusion with Thallium-201.

Angiographic Studies during the Attack
We were able to perform coronary arteriography during an anginal attack in 34 patients admitted to our C.C.U. because of frequent attacks of angina at rest usually of the "crescendo" type. The attack was spontaneous in 21 and induced by ergovine maleate intravenous injection in 17 (in 4 patients we performed coronary angiography both during a spontaneous and induced attack).

Resting coronary arteriography showed:
- normal vessels or only wall irregularities in 5 (all S-T elevation);
- 1 vessel disease (11 with S-T elevation, 2 with S-T depression);
- 2 vessels disease (7 with S-T elevation, 2 with S-T depression);
- 3 vessels disease (5 with S-T elevation, 2 with S-T depression).

In all patients with S-T segment elevation an occlusive diffuse vasospasm of the major coronary artery perfusing the myocardial territory corresponding to the ECG changes was observed. The finding was different only in degree (more or less diffuse) in the patients in whom it was observed during a spontaneous and induced attack (Figure 6). In patients with S-T segment depression, a spasm involving a small branch (Figure 7) or reducing collateral perfusion to one occluded branch or a diffuse reduction of vessel lumen without delayed filling and run off were observed (26).

Coronary spasm appears responsible for the hemodynamic pattern observed in these patients during the attack and for the reduced perfusion documented with Thallium-201 scintigraphy. The different location and extension of the spasm and the presence of collaterals may well account for the predominantly transmural or subendocardial distribution of ischemia. Thus "variant" or Prinzmetal angina (34) is only one extreme of a continuous spectrum of acute, transient myocardia ischemia with a transmural distribution caused by vasospasm. Lesser degrees of impairment of perfusion result in subendocardial ischemia. The observation of episodes of S-T segment elevation alternating with episodes of S-T segment depression in the same patient at few minutes distance in the same lead support this hypothesis (Figure 1).

Estimated Incidence of Vasospasm
The demonstrated existence of vasoconstriction as a factor controlling coronary blood supply requires a revision of the traditional assumption that the level of myocardial demand is the only determinant of the anginal threshold in the presence of coronary obstructions. Thus the possible existence of vasoconstriction can be suspected in all patients who appear to exhibit a wide variability of the anginal threshold, or present with angina at rest with preservation of exercise capacity.

Furthermore we have observed that "variant" angina, when appropriately searched for, may represent over 10% of patients with chest pain (35). If we accept that, with rare exceptions, "variant" angina may represent one of the landmarks of the syndrome of vasospastic angina, that vasospasm can also cause angina at rest with S-T segment depression and finally that under cold exposure (36) or exertion (37) vasoconstriction may be a precipitating factor for angina, the causal role of vasospasm in anginal patients appears to be much more frequent than generally thought.

Diagnostic and Therapeutic Implications

The demonstrated causal role of coronary vasospasm in the genesis of angina pectoris in the presence of a quite variable degree of coronary atherosclerotic lesions demands a careful diagnostic evaluation of anginal patients independently of the degree of coronary atherosclerotic obstructions observed at angiography.

The history of angina at rest with normal exercise tolerance, or angina on effort with a very variable threshold and with sometimes normal, maximal exercise tolerance may offer the first clue. Objective demonstration may be based on the absence of increased heart activity before the attack, on the reduction of myocardial perfusion, or on the angiographic observation of vasospasm during spontaneous attacks and possibly on the positivity of the ergonovine maleate test (38, 39) which, at the doses used in our laboratory, appears specific but not very sensitive (35).

As to the most direct therapeutic implications, in patients in whom vasospasm is recognized to be the only cause of angina neither betablockers, given with the purpose of lowering myocardial oxygen consumption, nor emergency by-pass coronary surgery appear to have a rational basis. For the time being, nitrates and calcium antagonists, which are known to vasodilate the large coronary arteries appear to be effective in reducing dramatically the number of attacks in these patients (40, 41).

REFERENCES

(1) Fothergill, J.M. (1879): The heart and its diseases. Lindsay and Blakison, Philadelphia.
(2) Osler, W. (1910): Lancet, 1, 702.
(3) Gallavardin, M.L. (1933): Lyon Med., 151, 217.
(4) Blumgart, H.L., Schlesinger, M.J. and Davis, D. (1940): Am. Heart J., 19, 1.
(5) Friedberg, L.K. (1966): Disease of the heart. 3rd Ed. Saunders Co., Philadelphia.
(6) Gianelly, R., Mugler, F. and Harrison, D.C. (1968): Calif. Med., 108, 129.
(7) Cheng, T.O., Bashour, T., Kelser, G.A., Jr., Weiss, L. and Bacos, J. (1973): Circulation, 47, 476.
(8) Bruschke, A.V.G., Proudfit, W.L. and Sones, F.M., Jr. (1973): Circulation, 47, 936.
(9) Kristian-Kerin, N., Davies, B. and Macleod, C.A. (1973): Chest, 64, 352.
(10) Guazzi, M., Polese, A., Fiorentini, C., Magrini, F. and Bartorelli, C. (1971): Br. Heart J., 33, 84.
(11) Maseri, A. (1976): "Primary" angina. 7th European Congress of Cardiology, Book II, p. 255.
(12) Dhurandhar, R.W., Watt, D.L., Silver, M.D., Trimble, A.S. and Adelman, A.G. (1972): Am. J. Cardiol., 30, 902.
(13) Froment, R., Normand, J. and Amiel, L. (1973): Arch. Mal. Coeur, 66, 755.
(14) Oliva, P.B., Potts, D.E. and Pluss, R.G. (1973): N. Engl. J. Med., 288, 745.
(15) Kerin, N. and Macleod, C.A. (1974): Br. Heart J., 36, 224.
(16) Conti, C.R., Brawley, R.K., Griffith, L.S.C., Pitt, B., Humphries, J.O., Gott, V.L. and Ross, R.S. (1973): Am. J. Cardiol., 32, 745.
(17) Fowler, N.O. (1972): Circulation, 46, 1079.
(18) Graybiel, A. (1955): U.S. Armed Forces Med. J., 6, 1.
(19) Chierchia, S., Maseri, A., Mimmo, R., Pesola, A. and Marchesi, C. (1975): Boll. Soc. Ital. Cardiol., 20, 931.
(20) Maseri, A., Pesola, A., Mimmo, R., Chierchia, S. and L'Abbate, A. (1975): Circulation, 52, Suppl. II, 89 (Abstract).
(21) Maseri, A., Mimmo, R., Chierchia, S., Marchesi, C., Pesola, A. and L'Abbate, A. (1975): Chest, 68, 625.
(22) Chierchia, S., Marchesi, C. and Maseri, A. (1977): International Workshop on "Angina Pectoris. Pathogenetic Mechanisms and Therapeutical Implications". Eds., Maseri, A., Klassen, G.A. and Lesch, M. Grune & Stratton, New York,

N.Y. (in press).

(23) Maseri, A., Parodi, O., Severi, S. and Pesola, A. (1976): Circulation, 54, 280.

(24) Parodi, O., Severi, S., Maseri, A., Biagini, A.,and Distante, A. (1977): International Workshop on "Angina Pectoris. Pathogenetic Mechanisms and Therapeutical Implications". Eds., Maseri, A., Klassen, G.A. and Lesch, M. Grune & Stratton, New York, N.Y. (in press).

(25) Pesola, A., Ballestra, A.M. and De Nes, D.M. (1977): International Workshop on "Angina Pectoris. Pathogenetic Mechanisms and Therapeutical Implications". Eds., Maseri, A., Klassen, G.A. and Lesch, M. Grune & Stratton, New York, N.Y. (in press).

(26) Maseri, A., L'Abbate, A., Pesola, A., Ballestra, A.M., Marzilli, M., Maltinti, G., Severi, S., De Nes, D.M., Parodi, O. and Biagini, A. (1977): Lancet, 1, 713.

(27) Bishop, V.S., Kaspar, R.L., Barnes, G.E. and Kardon, M.B. (1974): J. Apl. Physiol., 37, 785.

(28) Theroux, P., Ross, J., Franklin, D., Kemper, W. and Sasayama, S. (1976): Circulation, 53, 302.

(29) Heyndrickx, G.R., Millard, R.W., McRitchie, R.J., Maroko, P.R. and Vatner, S.F. (1975): J. Clin. Invest., 56, 978.

(30) Guazzi, M., Polese, A., Fiorentini, C., Magrini, F., Olivari, M.T. and Bartorelli, C. (1975): Brit. Heart J., 37, 401.

(31) Roughgarden, J.W. and Newman, E.V. (1966): Am. J. Med., 41, 935.

(32) Goldstein, R.E. and Epstein, S.E. (1972): Progr. Cardiovasc. Dis., 14, 360.

(33) Severi, S., Parodi, O., Maseri, A. and Solfanelli, S. (1977): XVI Congress of the Italian Society for Nuclear Biology and Medicine. (in press).

(34) Prinzmetal, M., Kennamer, R., Merliss, R., Wada, T. and Bor, N. (1959): Am. J. Med., 27, 375.

(35) Maseri, A., Chierchia, S., Severi, S. and Parodi, O. (1977): International Workshop on "Angina Pectoris. Pathogenetic Mechanisms and Therapeutical Implications". Eds., Maseri, A., Klassen, G.A. and Lesch, M. Grune & Stratton, New York, N.Y. (in press).

(36) Mudge, G.H., Grossman, W., Millis, R.M., Lesch, M. and Braunwald, E. (1976): N. Eng. J. Med., 295, 1333.

(37) Levene, D.L. and Freeman, M. (1976): J.A.M.A., 236, 1018.

(38) Clark, D.A., Quin, R.A., Bolen, J. and Schroeder, J.S. (1975): Am. J. Cardiol., 35, 127 (Abstract).

(39) Heupler, F., Proudfit, W., Siegel, W., Shirey, E., Razavi, M. and Sones, F.M. (1975): Circulation, 52, Suppl. II, 11.

(40) Distante, A., Severi, S., Biagini, A. and Maseri, A. (1977): International Workshop on "Angina Pectoris. Pathogenetic Mechanisms and Therapeutical Implications". Eds., Maseri, A., Klassen, G.A. and Lesch, M. Grune & Stratton, New York, N.Y. (in press).

(41) Parodi, O., Maseri, A., Simonetti, I., Chierchia, S., Severi, S. and L'Abbate, A.: Br. Heart J. (submitted for publication).

QUESTIONS

Dr. Jeremy Swan commented that these were very important demonstrations. He could quite visualize that, with a 30% organic lesion, spasm in the remaining wall could produce virtual or indeed complete obliteration of the lumen. Dr. Melvin Judkins did not contest the validity of the films shown by Dr. Maseri, but indicated his unhappiness to accept spasm in many of the angiograms submitted to him from other centres, for review.

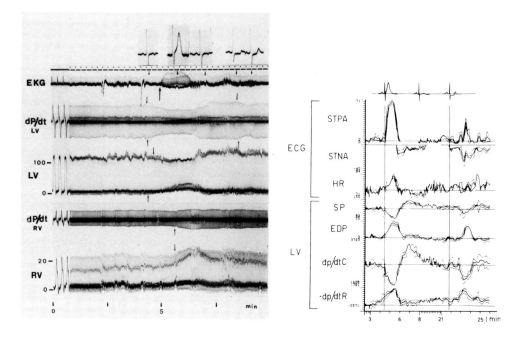

FIG. 1   A.   Low speed playback of a continuous recording of electrocardiographic
             lead V_4 (EKG), left and right ventricular (LV and RV) pressure and dp/
             dt. Two asymptomatic episodes of acute myocardial ischemia in rapid
             sequence can be observed.

         B.   The same episodes analysed by a computer (only ECG and LV parameters).
             The mean values at 10 seconds interval and their standard deviations
             are plotted with an expanded time scale during the episodes. STPA and
             STNA = S-T segment positive and negative areas. HR = heart rate; SP =
             systolic pressure dp/dt C and R = peak dp/dt of contraction and relax-
             ation phases (see text).

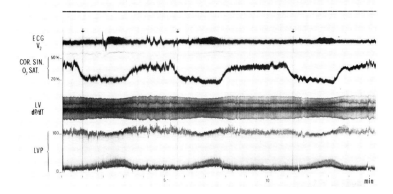

FIG. 2 Low speed play back of a continuous recording of left ventricular pressure
(LVP), dp/dt, coronary sinus oxygen saturation by a fiber-optic catheter
and ECG lead V_2. Three asymptomatic episodes of acute myocardial ischemia
with S-T segment elevation are visible (see text).

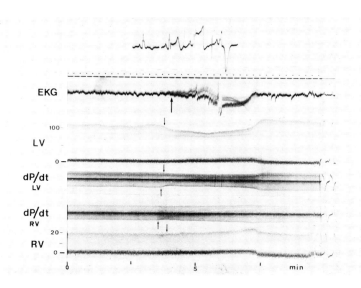

FIG. 3 Low speed play back of one episode of asymptomatic myocardial ischemia with
S-T segment changes in inferior leads. The reduction of relaxation dp/dt
is visible also in the right ventricular tracing suggesting also right
ventricular involvement by ischemia.

167

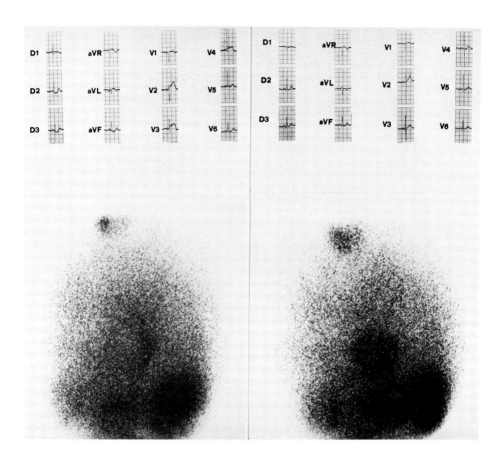

FIG. 4 A. Myocardial scintigram in LAC projection obtained following injection
           of Thallium-201 during angina at rest with S-T segment elevation induc-
           ed by ergonovine maleate. The ECG is at the top.

        B. Scintigram obtained a week later in the absence of signs of ischemia.
           A massive reduction of tracer uptake in the anterior wall and septum
           occurs during angina.

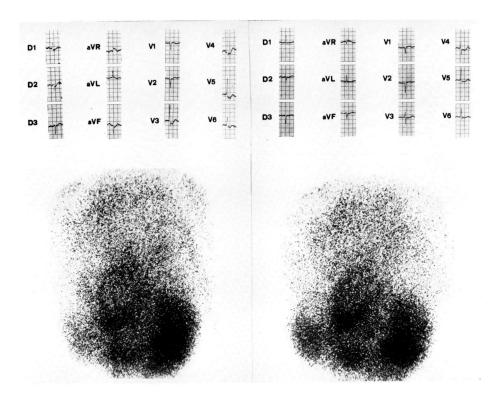

FIG. 5   A. Scintigram in LAO projection during spontaneous angina at rest with
              S-T segment depression.

          B. A week later in the absence of signs of ischemia. A reduced uptake
              which appears predominant in the anterior subendocardial regions is
              observed during angina.

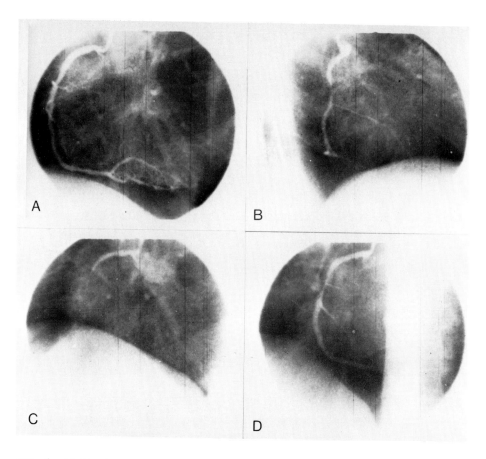

FIG. 6   Right cineangiography of a patient, A: in control (LAO projection), B:
during the very beginning of S-T segment elevation in the inferior leads
(RAO projection), C: during S-T segment elevation (LAO), D: during a
second anginal attack induced by ergonovine (LAO). The intensity of spasm
may vary in subsequent phases of the attack and in different attacks.

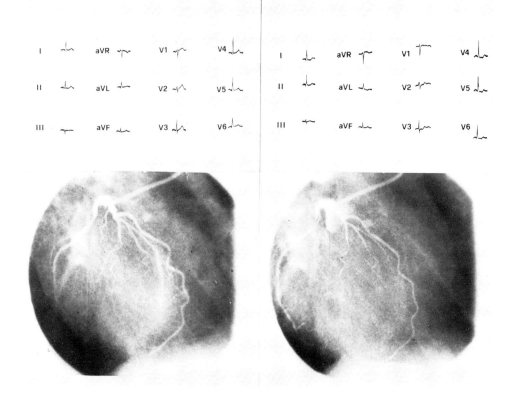

FIG. 7   Left coronary angiograms (RAO).

A.   During control.

B.   During spontaneous angina. The septal branch is very thin. It showed
     a marked delay in filling and run off.

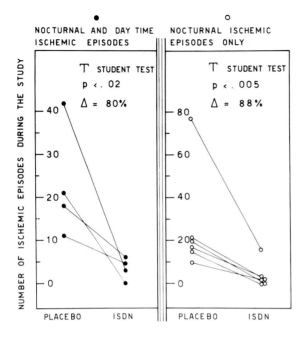

FIG. 8   Response to continuous infusion of isosorbide dinitrate (1.5 - 5 mg per
hour) versus placebo in a cross over study of 24 hour periods in 4 patients
(right), and of 12 hour periods in 6 patients (left) with angina at rest.

172

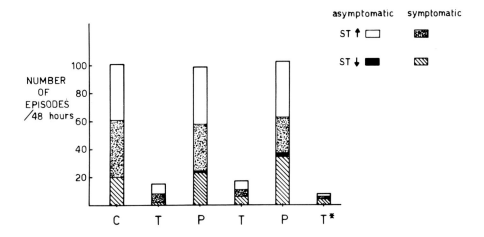

FIG. 9   Result of a double blind cross-over study with Verapamil of 48 hour periods
80 mg x 6 (T) and placebo (P) in patients with angina at rest in our C.C.U.
Continuing treatment for 2 days the end of the trial with 80 mg x 3 is
indicated by T*.

PANEL DISCUSSION ON THE DAY - May 5th

Chairman: Dr. Lawson McDonald

Speakers of the day joined by Dennis Krikler and Clive Layton

Dr. McDonald: (Light-hearted advice for Panel Discussions)
Professor Maseri, will you please answer the question about the possibility of
coronary spasm being induced by the catheter?

Professor Maseri: I have not much to say about it - I hoped that the film
could speak for itself. One of the last cases seen had the catheter in the
right coronary artery, and I thought what seemed to disappear was the diagonal
branch perfused by collaterals - that is quite a distance for a catheter-induc-
ed spasm. Secondly, I should like to be a statistician briefly and calculate
what is the probability - in millions or billions - of having a spasm during
the few injections when there are the ECG changes, but never in the several
hundred injections made in these patients when they have no ST segment changes.

(1) Dr. McDonald: I think you have really answered the question whether or not
spasm occurs at a distance from the catheter as well as close to the tip ...

Professor Maseri: I have no further comments about it.

(2) Dr. McDonald: How often does an asymptomatic person with a normal angiogram
show spasm after ergonovine?

Professor Maseri: I have no experience of this. As I said, I believe that the
ergonovine test is specific, but has low sensitivity at the doses we use, so
that we have never observed such effects. Usually, it is positive in patients
who say that they have several attacks a day ...

(3) Dr. McDonald: Is ergonovine safe?

Professor Maseri: Well, as with all tests, it depends on the way it is used.
It is important to be very careful, especially when experimenting with it. The
way we use it now has caused us no problems in over 230 patients.

(4) Dr. McDonald: The final question on the spasm problem is whether there is evidence of drugs other than nitrates which may influence spasm?

Professor Maseri: I have some slides on the subject, but did not have time to
show them. We have just completed a double-blind, crossover study with verapamil which shows impressive results. It will be published, so those interested can read about it.

Dr. Krikler: Do you see any reason why some people might be expected to react
adversely to β-blockers, as has been suggested by Japanese workers, in that
they may show spasm? Have you seen this in your experience?

Professor Maseri: I have no views about this because it is not our feeling
that this treatment is rational for these patients. We do not treat them with
β-blockers now. We used β-blockers before we became aware of the problem,

but I can recall the clinical impression - for what that is worth - that they increased the frequency of the attack. Another difference between us and the Japanese is that our patients do not respond to atropine. That is a mystery.

Professor Judkins: May I clarify one point made in my presentation - where I may have been misunderstood. I did not see a single film that I thought was not Prinzmetal's angina. What I said was in reference to cases sent to me - it is common for me to have cases sent with the query whether they are Prinzmetal's angina. The vast majority of them are clearly catheter-tip spasm right adjacent to the catheter tip - not this type of case, which is clearly Prinzmetal's angina. I have no disagreement with that.

(5) Question: What proportion of patients investigated in Professor Judkins' unit turn out to have normal coronary arteries, or trivial disease, and what is the effect of excluding these from his mortality figures?

Professor Judkins: My first thought is to give the percentage without arteriosclerotic obstructive disease. When we talk about normals, are we talking about absolute normals, people with normal coronary arteries but with a prolapsed valve producing their symptoms, or about valvular disease with or without coronary vessels affected? If all the normal coronary arteries are included, regardless of what other cardiac pathology the patients might have, we are talking about 20 per cent $\pm$ 2 per cent, according to which year we consider. The death rate at present is 0.05 per cent; over the past five years it has varied between 0.05 and 0.07 per cent. If we manipulate the figures, removing the 20 per cent normals, that still leaves a fairly low percentage.

What patients are those with whom we have trouble, that end up as fatalities? In general, these are the people with extremely bad ventricles. Three of our deaths have occurred in patients with proximally occluded anterior descending and proximally occluded right, and they were living on part of the circumflex system. These people do not pump well and if they are challenged slightly too much they are in trouble. That is the kind of patient at the highest risk in the laboratory.

Remember that we are dealing with a pressure-dependent system in this coronary artery disease. We are dealing with a non-compliant ventricle, and it is not very forgiving, so if it is over-challenged one way or another, there can rapidly be trouble, without much time to get out of that trouble.

(6) Dr. Layton: Dr. Erikssen (Oslo) disagrees strongly with Professor Judkins so perhaps he will pose his question, or problem, himself.

Dr. Erikssen: I completely disagree with the $t_{\frac{1}{2}}$ given by Professor Judkins for his obstructions - if I remember correctly, he said that there was a $t_{\frac{1}{2}}$ of 1.3 years. In our paper, reported yesterday by Dr. Coltart, we now have about $3\frac{1}{2}$ years follow-up on our angiographed asymptomatic males. There have been no myocardial infarctions, nor a single case of angina, all the men are at work and are well. Most of these men had had at least one obstruction of 75 per cent.

Professor Judkins: This reminds me again of this iceberg. It seems incredible that in coronary disease we can produce completely different figures from subsets which do not seem to be very different. What is worse, we can look at the same subsets and still come up with different figures. In Dr. Erikssen's subset, the patients were all non-symptomatic, picked up by stress testing - they were not at the critical stage. Perhaps we are measuring percentages in different ways, but Dr. Erikssen's patients were non-symptomatic, whereas my subset

were people basically with progressive angina and who were symptomatic, thus
further along in their disease. I do not know why the figures show such a
discrepancy. Our figures are taken from one year's consecutive cases in whom
there was over 80 per cent stenosis in a vessel. The follow-up was angiographic in about one-third of the patients. In the remainder, there was clinical
follow-up: the referring physician sent us a card to say the patient had died,
indicating whether or not as a result of a myocardial infarction, or to say
that the patient had had a myocardial infarction during the period of observation.

This was not an absolute follow-up: there may be more registered infarcts than
we appeared to have because we did not have angiographic follow-up on them all.
In the angiographic group about one-third fell into the same range as the patients about whom we just had a card reply from the referring physician. I
think the results were reasonably reliable - but it was a subset of symptomatic
patients.

Dr. Krikler: I think that Professor Judkins made a most convincing case for
having the totality of the information available before making therapeutic
decisions. I wonder whether this does not include the need to have the sort of
functional assessment implicit in Professor Maseri's studies, excluding people
with extensive three-vessel disease. Do you not think that in people with two-
vessel, or the minority you see with one-vessel disease additional stress testing, implicit in, say, the use of ergonovine, might be helpful? Might this not
perhaps show those patients who are unsuitable for surgery, or alternatively
should have a different medical method considered? Might this sort of case
perhaps help to explain the varying incidence of patients - perhaps 10 to 20
per cent - who develop Q waves, or other signs of post-bypass, post-surgical
infarction?

Professor Judkins: The answer to that question is obvious: the better we work
up a patient the better results we will have because we will be able to select
a better therapy. If ergonovine studies were done on all our patients, we
might gain a little additional information. However, the ergonovine study is
early. Although it has been advocated by some, other people object rather viol-
ently to this as an accurate and safe test.

We have used this test, always with a great deal of caution because it is easy
to get into trouble with it. It should not be used without having the appropriate drugs and so on available in order to counteract the effect.

Dr. McDonald: I have two questions of extreme importance, which I will put to
the whole Panel. First, what is the origin of pain in the heart?

Professor Maseri: I do not have the slightest idea where pain comes from, but
what is important is that when it occurs it is a late phenomenon, not an indicator of the onset of ischaemia generally. It can be absent during severe ischaemia; it is possible to have severe arrhythmias with ventricular tachycardia
during one of these attacks of variant, or non-variant angina without pain, the
patient passing away very gently.

Dr. McDonald: Would anyone like to enlarge on the origin of pain in the heart?

Dr. Swan: Chatterjee's studies a few years ago showed clearly that lactate in
high concentrations in the coronary sinus does not necessarily result in pain.
Thus, pain does not appear to be absolutely dependent on lactate production.
It is clear, too, that pain is a highly variable phenomenon, not necessarily
occurring in large-territory ischaemia but occurring equally well in small-
territory ischaemia. There is no direct relationship between pain and the

magnitude of the ischaemia. There are, of course, nerve fibres - poorly studied - in the human heart. Many potentially experimental species cannot report the presence of pain but, if there are conscious animal preparations in whom either coronary constriction, or indeed pulmonary artery occlusion is generated by artificial means, the animals become distressed. If they are in the running phase of their activity, they will stop, they will have gastrointestinal upsets which are unpleasant for all concerned - front end and rear. It appears that some major, central phenomena are going on which might be suggestive of the particular phenomenon of pain.

One of the problems here is that the nerve supply of the heart is not thoroughly understood; the presence of pain receptors is not described, to my knowledge.

(8) Dr. McDonald: That answer has partially anticipated the next question on the same theme: what is the sensory innervation of the heart, what and where are the pain receptors? Perhaps Professor Harris might have something to say on this topic? ... (Professor Harris has no comment to make) ... I am thus forced to the interesting conclusion that this Meeting neither knows the source of pain in the heart nor how it travels - if it starts in the heart - to where the patient feels it. Professor Pitt, would that be the view at Johns Hopkins?

Professor Pitt: I do not think that anyone has any firm data. Some of the most promising clues, however, may be from the prostaglandins and bradykinin systems. Several years ago we showed that in human angina pectoris there is a variable bradykinin release. More recently, the St. Louis group has shown the relationships of bradykinin to prostaglandins. The assays are extremely difficult, but this avenue, of all the possibilities, looks perhaps the most promising. No one, of course, has any final data yet.

(9) Dr. Layton: A question from Dr. Wainwright (London) - The separation of uptake defects into perfusion and metabolic components may be important in the investigation of patients with normal coronary arteries and abnormal myocardial lactate production. Is it possible to estimate the relative contribution of these components to uptake defects with ^{13}N ...?

Professor Resnekov: I think that the answer is "no" at present. We are leading towards investigations in that direction. I certainly agree about its potential importance. As I indicated in my presentation, there are agents which will look particularly at perfusion without any metabolic component to it. Presumably, a combination study will enable us to tell the difference between an uptake defect, which is primarily related to perfusion, and the other type which may or may not be related to some metabolic abnormality.

Dr. Layton: Dr. Wainwright goes on to suggest that there might be some benefit in comparing early and delayed images after a single dose of ^{13}N.

Professor Resnekov: That is certainly a possibility. As is well-known, there have been studies of this sort using thallium, looking at it immediately after the injection and about six hours later. We do not have this particular problem with the ^{13}NH$_4$ scan since its half-life is sufficiently short for us to repeat the studies as often as we wish.

Dr. Layton: The second part of the same question by Dr. Wainwright was whether you have any information on uptake defects in the particular group of patients - that is, in those with normal coronary arteries and abnormal myocardial lactate production?

Professor Resnekov: Yes, we have seen it in a variety of groups of patients.

s. One such group, interestingly, is this strange syndrome described by Professor Barlow, on which he might like to comment: in prolapse of the mitral valve a group of patients have angina pectoris clinically, they produce lactate on stressing the heart in one way or another, and uptake defects can readily be demonstrated by these techniques. We have also seen it in the cardiomyopathic group, both the congestive and obstructive varieties, as well as in other situations in which we believe there is no clinical evidence of the presence of disease. Although this technique is very useful in the presence of known disease, there remains much to be learnt about its specificity and sensitivity in a wide variety of situations.

Dr. McDonald: Professor Pitt, would you like to comment on those questions?

Professor Pitt: In answer to the second question, we have studied a fairly large group of patients with normal coronary arteries, looking at two "subgroups". In the first, volunteers - usually fellow physicians, house officers and nurses - no false positives were found. In the second group, patients with normal coronary arteries who have presented with atypical chest pain, we have found some with perfusion defects - whether they are false positives, or what they mean, we are not in a position to decide. Finding a positive perfusion defect in this group is an indication that we should go further and do some more sophisticated metabolic studies. It is probably a clue suggesting that the patients are not being followed as well as they should be.

Professor Resnekov: There is one technical problem that we encounter in which I am sure we see false positives. I would be interested to hear Professor Pitt's view about it. This is usually found in young, normal volunteers again,

apical region
uptake defect

in which the apical region of the heart is being investigated. Very frequently, we see what appears to be an uptake defect in that apical region. I suspect that the reason relates to the motion of the heart and the rapidity of beating. If there is a tachycardia, this is seen much more frequently than if there is not. This apical region of the ventricle is a region in which I believe we can be led astray, and where the incidence of false positives is higher than in the other regions of the heart, particularly in younger people.

Professor Pitt: It is important to be extremely conservative about the interpretation of perfusion defects at the apex. Motion may be one thing, but the anatomy is perhaps more important. If we look carefully at the anatomy of the muscle, the thickness of the myocardium at the apex is perhaps 20 per cent of the thickness in the free wall, so we will see perfusion defects there. Thus, we must be conservative about interpreting a perfusion defect in the apex. If there is a clear cut-off, sharp and very discrete, we call it abnormal, but we frequently see a perfusion defect in the normals. It is a matter of how these things are interpreted, but I think that there is an anatomic reason.

Dr. McDonald: We are pleased to have Professor Barlow here from Johannesburg. As we all know, he is professor of the posterior cusp problem, which has made us all look in more detail at a number of patients in relation to their pain. Perhaps he can give us his latest views on the source of pain in such people - these patients with prolapsed posterior cusp?

Professor Barlow: It would be nice if I had something meaningful to say about it. We think there are two forms of pain: first, the typical angina - typical in site, although not typical in behaviour, in response to effort or emotion - and secondly, the atypical fleeting chest pain which is often left-sided and not necessarily related to emotion or to exercise. I do not know the cause of these pains. The more typical angina may be related to coronary artery spasm. There is some reason to suspect an association in some instances between coronary artery spasm and prolapse of the mitral valve. The atypical pain may be due to traction on the papillary muscles - I have no other suggestion about its cause.

(10) Dr. McDonald: The first question for Professor Julian may have been partially covered, but it is relevant to the title of this Meeting: how often are conduction disturbances, or a dysrhythmia the first feature in an otherwise asymptomatic patient?

Professor Julian: I do not know the answer to that question. Certainly, a bundle branch block can be the first feature sometimes, although I should not like to say how often. I think it is in only a small percentage of cases. Someone else can probably answer the question better than I can.

Dr. Krikler: It is likely that the percentage in which it is a first feature is fairly small if it is an isolated finding. This can be taken into account with longevity studies which have shown that many of these people have developed - or shown - such phenomena incidentally at insurance, or other examinations. Many good illustrations of this appeared in the days of electrocardiography, as reported by Dr. Paul White in his book "Heart: the long follow-up". There were many such asymptomatic individuals with follow-up periods of 30 to 40 years, some of them developing manifestations of ischaemic heart disease of a more classical nature after perhaps 20 years - when it might be expected in any case.

Professor Julian: This has been confirmed by Kulbertus' study in Belgium, in which he carried out many community reviews on ECGs, looking particularly for manifestations of bundle branch block. The phenomena which we think are such highly significant and dangerous events after infarction have an astonishingly good prognosis.

(11) Dr. Layton: A question from Dr. Dienstl (Innsbruck) - we have observed a few cases of relatively young men who have died suddenly during physical exercise who have showed haemorrhagic pneumonia. Does Professor Julian think that these cases could belong to the sudden death group of an infectious, possibly viral, aetiology?

(12) Secondly (from Dr. Schwartz), how important, if at all, is myocarditis in the sudden death syndrome?

Professor Julian: This is a greatly under-studied subject. We are probably missing quite a lot of these because they seldom have viral studies - it is not easy to carry out viral studies. About two weeks ago I saw a Coxsackie myocarditis presenting as an acute infarct with enzyme changes. Coronary angiography showed the coronary arteries to be entirely normal. I suspect it is far more common than we realise and that it forms a significant proportion of sudden deaths, particularly in that group of exercising athletes who die during, or after physical exercise.

(13) Dr. Layton: (from Dr. A.D. Levine (Oakland, California)) - Could you discuss the problem of treating a patient with antiarrhythmic agents in the light of their myocardial depressant effects, especially in view of your comments on

ventricular dysfunction and sudden death?

Professor Julian: I am not sure that it is not outside the scope of this Meeting. Some of the newer antiarrhythmic drugs, such as mexiletine, disopyramide, tocanide, aprinidine and so on, have much less myocardial depressant effect than, for example, quinidine, procainamide and the β-blockers. I am not too sure about disopyramide because I have seen some cases of pulmonary oedema occurring in patients with poor left ventricular function who are put on to disopyramide. I have not seen this happen with our very short experience with tocanide or with mexiletine. I think, therefore, that I am prepared to give these drugs to patients with poor left ventricular function. In many of these cases I am more worried about the possibility of inducing conduction defects, in those who already have some degree of conduction abnormality. I do not think that left ventricular dysfunction is a strong contraindication for the more modern antiarrhythmic drugs.

(14) Dr. Krikler: A question from Dr. Massoud (Paris) - This question relates to Dr. Swan's interesting technique which he presented today. What are the repercussions likely to be in the future as a result of applying his method using CKG in the assessment of left ventricular function, as regards the surgical indications, say for coronary bypass for these patients? In other words, would he advise an operation on these patients at this early stage of detection, before further deterioration of left ventricular myocardial function, or does he prefer to advise medical treatment and follow up using this technique, later on deciding about surgery?

Dr. Swan: I do not think we are able at this time to define appropriately the treatment of the asymptomatic patient, or the patient who does not present with overt coronary disease with clear-cut symptoms. The purpose of my presentation today was to identify those patients who were more likely to have important myocardial ischaemia and, by inference, the possibility in a high proportion of cases of coronary arterial disease. I do not think that we are in any position to recommend therapy on this basis. I believe, as Dr. Kottke said yesterday, that we have to make a diagnosis - we are not making diagnoses sufficiently early. Once we do that, we can start on different treatment regimens, depending upon the specifics of an individual patient group.

The implication, of course, is that this will turn up many more patients and will, therefore, present at risk a great number of patients to surgery or to surgeons. This is not implicit at all, I believe, in what we have been talking about.

(15) Dr. McDonald: Dr. Bruyneel (Antwerp) has come to our rescue on the question about the origin of pain. This is a question which we have been asking ourselves: whether or not after cardiac transplantation the patients have true angina pectoris. We know that they develop occlusive arterial disease, but do they get true angina pectoris? Those in London did not, but Dr. Bruyneel has some first-hand information on Professor Barnard's cases.

Dr. Bruyneel: First, I have only limited experience on a few cases - the ones who survived! Professor Barnard's second patient developed extensive coronary sclerotic disease in his second heart, also angina pectoris. Another case, much later on, is doing very well, developing angina only on a cycling ergometer. He can manage during normal life, but develops angina pectoris under heavy exercise showing that a denervated system is not important for the development of angina - because it is developed quite early if the patients are exercised about two months after transplantation. The other case that I mentioned was exercised about six weeks after transplantation - it was early because he was recovering very well ...

Dr. McDonald: (intervening) In effect, this was a denervated heart?

Dr. Bruyneel: Yes - it was total transplantation ...

Dr. McDonald: That is the first point that ought to be made.

Dr. Bruyneel: Total innervation seems to be less important for the development of angina pectoris than some sort of metabolic origin.

Dr. McDonald: Whereabouts was the pain in this patient you have described? The distribution of angina pectoris is known to us all - where did he experience pain?

Dr. Bruyneel: In the chest - he had retrosternal pain and shortness of breath.

Dr. McDonald: Dr. Moret, you are a metabolic doctor - have you any comment on this subject? ... (Dr. Moret (Geneva) had no comment to make)

(16) Dr. McDonald: Professor Maseri, is spasm sex-linked? I am not sure what that means!

Professor Maseri: I hope it means in relation to being male or female. Most of our patients are male.

Dr. Krikler: There are two questions covering rather similar ground - one of the points has already been raised.

(17) Dr. Van de Sande (Antwerp) asks - If my impression is right, women more often have the symptomatology of myocardial infarction with a normal coronary arteriogram. Can this be explained entirely by the use of the Pill, or can other factors come into play, whether they be smoking or hormonal?

(18) and Dr. Ruttley (Cardiff) - We have had a rash of youngish women with atypical chest pain and normal coronaries, not provoked by ergot. Pregnancy has a high incidence in young women (Dr. Krikler - a reasonable statement) and ergotamine is used in labour. Do people see spasm referred from the labour wards?

Dr. Layton: In answer to the last part of the question, when we started to use ergonovine - ergometrine in our case - we discovered that migraine clinics in this country which prescribed ergotamine to their patients frequently told them not to worry if they experienced chest pain as a result of this treatment. It is apparently a well-recognised phenomenon among people who have used the drug extensively.

Professor Maseri: In the 1950s there were a number of papers in the American Heart Journal and other journals about ergonovine which at that time was proposed as a test for angina in a general sense. There were tracings in these articles, the author of which I cannot remember, showing ST segment depression following much higher doses of ergonovine. There are cases reported in the literature of people treated for migraine with ergonovine who developed myocardial infarction, angina and so on. All these reports were in the 1950s. That is all I know about it.

Professor Resnekov: I will not comment on the question, but will make an anecdotal observation which I think is a real one. We are seeing an increasing amount of true myocardial infarction, with true coronary atherosclerosis in younger women. I have thought about this and wonder whether it is a consequence of the Women's Lib movement in that women are now having to perform as housewives and mothers and all the other marvellous things they do, but also in the

ordinary market place, in the professions and so on. It is enormously difficult these days to be a woman.

Dr. McDonald: Professor Pitt, what is the answer in Baltimore? ... (Professor
Pitt had no comment to make) Professor Judkins, can you tell us the answer?

Professor Judkins: The way I understood the original question it asked whether
there is a sex relationship between true myocardial infarcts and normal coronary arteries. In our experience, it is something of a toss-up. We see true
myocardial infarcts both in men and women, perhaps slightly favouring men as
far as numbers are concerned - a higher number in men - but not predominantly
one or the other. This has nothing to do with Prinzmetal's disease, but just
infarcts without recognisable obstructions. From what I said earlier, it
should have been sensed that I do not believe that most of these people have
not had an obstruction. There is a certain amount of evidence that many of
these people have had an obstruction which probably caused their infarct, but
that that obstruction is no longer evident by the time they are studied.

(19) Dr. McDonald: There has been quite a lot of mention today about sudden death
in relation to left ventricular dysfunction. Clearly, the two are closely related. If we pursue that line of thought slightly further, do they always go
together? I should like to hear the views of the Panel about it. Is there
electrophysiological instability which may be totally independent of left
ventricular dysfunction as we measure it? Dr. Swan initiated this line of
thought this morning, so perhaps he could comment?

Dr. Swan: Professor Julian should answer that question. The issue of sudden
death and ventricular dysfunction is, in general, in those patients with clear-
cut, evident coronary artery disease. They comprise a substantial fraction of
those patients who have sudden death. They are frequently late phenomena in
the disease entity itself. Ventricular dysfunction is not necessarily present
in the great majority of those patients whose first cardiac event is a "sudden
death" with or without resuscitation. Dr. Bruce indicated - certainly, it has
been our finding - that in patients with very severe coronary disease who are
resuscitated fast it is possible to demonstrate completely normal cardiac function at a point in time slightly down stream.

As far as death and cardiac dysfunction are concerned: global myocardial failure can occur if there is a degree of reduction in the relative volume of blood
reaching the heart muscle. This becomes a very rapidly progressive vicious
cycle and may account for the five to ten minute death as opposed to the instantaneous cardiac death. These are the patients with the acute symptoms.
Remember that it is impossible to have a myocardial infarction in five minutes:
that muscle is not dead in five minutes, no cells of that muscle are dead in
that time, but the patient can be dead in five minutes because of global cardiac
dysfunction.

My answer to the question is that it is true that sudden death occurs in very
bad coronary disease, but that sudden death can occur as a first event in serious coronary disease without necessarily overt previous ventricular dysfunction
having been present.

Professor Julian: I agree with Dr. Swan's remarks. We have to differentiate
between these post-infarct patients, in whom manifest left ventricular dysfunction is a very important factor in their sudden death, and individuals who have
apparently been in good health and who drop dead suddenly. Many of us know
friends and relations in whom the latter has happened. A friend of mine a
couple of weeks ago played a vigorous game of squash, sat down afterwards and

while talking dropped down dead. He was found to have a three-vessel disease at post-mortem - he was not resuscitated successfully unfortunately.

Leonard Cobb, in his study on resuscitated ventricular fibrillation patients has shown that one in three has single-vessel disease, one in three two-vessel disease and one in three has three-vessel disease, with half the patients having ejection fractions greater than 50 per cent. Of course, it has to be borne in mind that these are resuscitated patients and are not a complete spectrum of all patients who have ventricular fibrillation. The fact that they are resuscitated may mean that they are relatively mild. Quite a substantial proportion of these patients do not have very advanced coronary arterial disease nor advanced left ventricular dysfunction. Undoubtedly, it is an important factor, but certainly not the only one.

Professor Pitt: When we talk about the relationship of left ventricular dysfunction to sudden death we may be oversimplifying matters. I cannot comment on the sudden death in the asymptomatic patients, but I should like to describe some of our experience in sudden death in patients post-myocardial infarction. We have now angiogrammed about 100 patients two weeks after myocardial infarction, following them up and looking at the subsequent sudden deaths. If we look only at overall left ventricular dysfunction, there is certainly a relationship - but that is too gross and too simple. If we investigate patients who have had an infarct in a completely akinetic area, regardless of whether they have a low ejection fraction of less than 40 per cent, or one above 40 per cent they have an excellent prognosis. However, if the patient has a hypokinetic area served by a narrowed vessel, that is the sort of patient who goes on to sudden death, to future myocardial infarction and to chest pain following myocardial infarction.

Dr. McDonald: Regarding electrophysiological instability and ventricular dysfunction, have either Professor Blankenhorn or Dr. Bruce any further comments about it?

Dr. Bruce: There are some interesting disparities in our clinical observations. Once again, to refer to those 17 cases involved in exercise which I mentioned as unpredictable, psychogenic factors may well have been important precipitating events in two of them. In one case, the patient was starting to jog around the gym floor, with his personal physician in attendance - next to him, doing the same thing - they started talking about heart disease, particularly the problems of sudden cardiac arrest, and in the next lap he suddenly said he did not feel well. Fortunately, he was near the defibrillator, the paddles were put on and the ECG was visualised immediately - he had sudden cardiac arrest with VF. Another patient, in this same series of 17, had a sudden cardiac arrest one minute after another patient had fallen to the floor and was in the process of being resuscitated. The second patient came around, saw the first one being resuscitated, he fell to the floor. There are many factors involved, and I suggest the possibility of psychogenic stimuli, however mediated, being the important factor at that moment. Whatever it is that is critical to any given individual is also unpredictable until afterwards when it can be thought about in retrospect.

Another disparity is that the first man of these 17 patients - who, like the majority of these individuals, has continued in the programme after being observed in coronary care for three to five days after infarction - has continued for seven years in the same training programme, three mornings a week, with no complaints and no recurrence. This stands in vivid contrast to the experience in the general community in which at least 30 per cent of these people have a recurrence of VF within the first year - and die of it, even though the fire department usually responds. This raises the other question of how much of this is simply a random event superimposed on the substrate of severe coronary disease in 90 to 95 per cent of the cases? This still leaves a very small fraction who cannot be explained even on that basis.

I can describe one other anecdotal experience about a young athlete, a 28-year-old football coach. He was apparently in perfect health, but he dropped down on the playing field. The fire department resuscitated him from VF. That same evening he had a recurrence and could not be resuscitated. At autopsy he had entirely normal coronary arteries, myocardium and valves - there was no suggestion of anything. Finally, on serial sectioning, he was found to have a single, focal, macrocytic infiltrative lesion. The pathologist, from his experience, stated that such an histological appearance meant that the man must have had a focal lesion for at least ten days. That is all that was ever found - but he was just as dead as all the others.

Professor Blankenhorn: I have nothing to add - I am not sure whether I want to stand up and talk too long about the subject after hearing those two stories. One philosophical comment, however, is that all of these concepts should be age-corrected. My personal view is that at some ripe old age - I am currently naming it at 90 - I hope to die suddenly.

Dr. McDonald: Perhaps that old friend of British cardiology, Dr. Selzer, would like to comment?

Dr. Selzer (San Francisco): In relation to sudden death, I have always wondered whether we are putting too many different things together. Is it a coronary death in a patient who dies suddenly and who has coronary disease, or could it be an electrical death in patients who happen to have anatomic changes in the coronary arteries? There is a great need to subdivide and identify subsets which are definitely due to ischaemia triggering death, as distinct from deaths from many other causes. We have already discussed the prolapsing mitral valve, hypertrophic cardiomyopathy - there are many causes of sudden death which are usually all put together as though they were a single entity.

Dr. Krikler: Excluding your own subjects, where do the members of the Panel think they see the greatest progress likely to come in the very early recognition of coronary artery disease, after the two days' discussions? (Professor Judkins asks for time to think about the question)

Professor Maseri: The history.

Dr. Swan: I think that the recognition of the possibility of spasm - this has no connection with Professor Maseri's favourite point - is something which should now be explored further. What Professor Maseri did not say was that coronary arteries as biological phenomena in certain individuals in the operating room, are exquisitely sensitive to stimuli. At the first touch of a scalpel on those vessels in certain patients, there is a contraction in a most complete manner. If we can visualise a small coronary lesion, with 30 per cent occlusion, of which 70 per cent of the wall is muscle, a spasm in that vessel on that lesion could give rise to many of the problems we have been discussing.

Professor Julian: I should like to support Professor Maseri on the history, except to go further and say that we should be more aggressive about looking for the history. One of the fascinating stories Professor Judkins told us was about the patient with angina ten years previously - he must have had the 80 per cent stenosis ten years previously and, if action had been taken at that time, the story might have been a happier one. The history side needs to be pushed much harder.

Professor Resnekov: I should like to see a much firmer interrelationship between all the aspects about which we have been talking at this Meeting. We tend to look at the subject from our own particular vantage point, but I believe in a disease so multifactorial as the one we are discussing we need to concentrate heavily on putting together all our information. Once that has been done, some of these unsolved questions will indeed be answered.

Professor Pitt: Over the next few years, with some of the newer, non-invasive techniques, it should be possible to have an earlier detection of anatomic coronary artery disease through functional testing. There are several approaches to this, all of them in their infancy. Perhaps we will never be able to get early enough, but we should be able to pick up some of the patients with significant coronary artery disease by means of functional testing.

Dr. McDonald: Professor Judkins, if you would prefer to show us again that wonderful picture of the geese, rather than say any more, we would be content to leave it at that. (Professor Judkins has packed the picture away)

Professor Judkins: The fundamental problem here in the early recognition of coronary disease is to recognise the patient who is potentially a victim of ischaemic heart disease. We have to go to the history. As has been indicated earlier this afternoon, our best percentage chance of picking up people with ischaemic heart disease, in whom these various tests can be done, is for an aware physician to recognise the possibility. Other physicians need to be better educated in the early recognition of coronary disease, principally by the history.

Dr. McDonald: Thank you very much. I should like to thank all members of the Panel for answering the questions with such remarkable ability. (Applause)

SUMMARY

Leon Resnekov

Important points brought out during the course of the two day meeting can be summarised as follows:-

Population Studies
There is a great need for further studies in children and young adolescents to determine factors of importance in the subsequent development of coronary heart disease. Professor Walter Holland reported on studies in children of various social
classes to detect blood pressure abnormalities, smoking habits and body size. Con-
cern was also expressed about the possible deleterious effects of the use of contraceptive pills by adolescent girls.

Whereas a great deal of effort has been extended on population studies documenting
normal and abnormal lipid patterns, Dr. Joan Slack indicated the need for selective
screening of levels of blood pressure, total cholesterol and smoking habits. Such
selective screening aimed at uncovering groups of patients at particular risk are
more likely to be beneficial than non-selective mass screening programs.

Thrombosis and Platelet Function
Professor Tony Mitchell indicated that up to the present no test of platelet function is available for widespread field application. Furthermore, all tests currently
used are extravascular whereas additional information of importance might well result from intravascular studies which whilst desirable, are not as yet available.

Genesis of Atherosclerosis
Dr. Colin Schwartz summarised present views regarding the causes and formation of
atherosclerotic arterial lesions and indicated that abnormalities of endothelial
permeability in very young animals occurred at sites which were predestined for the
formation of atherosclerotic lesions. There is an important interaction between the
proliferation of smooth muscle cells and lipoproteins in the development of the lesion. Much of the experimental work reported by Dr. Schwartz was undertaken in very
young animals - again emphasising the need for investigations clinically in the
paediatric age group in which the atherosclerotic process might well commence.

Sudden Death
This topic was discussed by Professor Desmond Julian. There seems no true definition of "sudden death", a fatality within 24 hours of an acute cardiac event often
being labelled as such. Amongst premonitory signs can be included fatigue and chest
pain. The actual event may be precipitated by sudden unaccustomed effort, by acute
psychological factors and even by acute infections, sometimes viral in origin. Perhaps rapid retrieval systems in communities offer the best hope of dealing with the
problem, if not of preventing it.

Exercise Testing
Drs. John Coltart and Robert Bruce presented information about exercise testing.
The sensitivity and specificity of all such testing needs to be known but also has
to be compared with the prevalence of the disease being investigated in the population under survey. Dr. Bruce indicated that the predictive value of exercise testing

was enhanced by the development of cardiac pain during the test, particularly if associated with significant ST segment depression on the electrocardiogram. Equally important, however, was the functional capacity of the patient. Heart rate impairment when exercising to maximal effort and an abnormal blood pressure response were both of great value. Considering the enormity of the task, if exercise testing is to be applied to large groups, Dr. Bruce suggested that these tests might be used under two different circumstances:-

1. In those in whom risk factors for the development of coronary heart disease are present, exercising to maximal (not submaximal) capability to help identify individuals at particular risk.

2. Exercise testing without prior screening might be used alternatively to identify a high risk group incapable of exercising for six minutes because of cardiac limitation.

Newer Techniques

Amongst non-invasive techniques of use not only in demonstrating, but also in quantitating arteriosclerotic lesions in large peripheral arteries, Dr. David Blankenhorn described a novel method for the quantitative assessment angiographically of lesions in the femoral artery. Dr. Bruce Kottke discussed the role of high resolution ultrasound in demonstrating and sizing lesions of the carotid arteries. This method has a resolution of 1 - 2 mm.

Although these approaches are as yet not suitable for investigating the coronary circulation, their potential importance in arteriosclerotic disease is their ready applicability particularly for studying regression of arteriosclerotic lesions.

Two techniques were described which assess left ventricular function. Dr. Jeremy Swan discussed a new method of cardiokymography in which information about ventricular wall motion is obtained non-invasively and which can be used to demonstrate segmental left ventricular dysfunction. The method is inexpensive and can be repeated for sequential studies. In its present form it is non-linear and further development and refinement of the technique will be undertaken to assess its possible role in the early detection of coronary heart disease. Dr. Derek Gibson discussed the use of echocardiography as a measure of segmental and total ventricular function and showed examples of computer analysed echocardiograms to demonstrate and localise abnormalities of left ventricular contractions.

Myocardial Imaging

Two presentations were devoted to the use of cardiac imaging. Dr. Bertram Pitt in the 1977 Haile Selassie Lecture, discussed the use of "cold spot" imaging following an injection of 201-Thallium to determine myocardial uptake defects, "hot spot" imaging using 99m-Technetium Pyrophosphate to demonstrate myocardial infarction and acute ischemia and gated blood pool scintigraphy as a measure of regional and total ventricular function.

Dr. Leon Resnekov presented information about the use of short half-lived positron emitting nuclides manufactured in an on-site cyclotron for myocardial gamma-camera scintigraphic uptake (cold spot) imaging applicable to the very ill patient. Because of its short half-life repeated and sequential imaging studies can be done in safety. The nuclide nitrogen-13 as ammonia can also be imaged using a novel double camera system for positron imaging of the heart. Computer handling of the data from the two cameras is used to develop any number of desired back projection tomographic images of the myocardium thus providing accurate anatomical localisation of uptake defects and the possibility of sizing the lesions and quantitating the information.

Coronary Arteriography

Dr. Melvin Judkins discussed the use of coronary arteriography and left ventriculography to demonstrate lesions of the coronary arteries and their effect on left
ventricular function. Up to the present no other technique is capable of providing
the anatomical information of these diagnostic methods.

Dr. Attilio Maseri discussed the significance of coronary artery spasm in the pre-
cipitation of cardiac pain and demonstrated its frequency and importance in the
overall symptomatology of coronary heart disease and particularly in syndromes such
as unstable angina pectoris.

Whereas it is apparent that no single test is capable of documenting the presence
of coronary heart disease, particularly when asymptomatic, a graduated diagnostic
approach seems appropriate. Starting with a careful history and physical examination, risk subsets in relation to blood pressure, smoking habits, body size and
lipids are then defined. Thereafter exercise testing and the non-invasive tests of
myocardial function including isotopic imaging and echocardiography are performed
to document patients at particular risk. In those in whom high risk is established,
coronary arteriography and left ventriculography can be used to demonstrate the presence of the lesions and their effect on regional and total ventricular function.

The two days of the meeting brought to light much additional information, but also
surprising gaps in our overall knowledge. Very little was heard about electro-
physiology and there was clearly room for greater inter-related studies. Further
work is needed on demonstrating mechanical dysfunction of the ventricle as an early
marker of disease. In addition, many of the speakers, particularly answering questions during the panels, indicated the possible importance of psychological factors
yet no definite statement could be made about this aspect at the present time. The
importance of population studies in the paediatric age group needs to be emphasised.

Further efforts are needed in setting up programmes of prevention, combining groups
of physicians, sociologists and psychologists.

As a whole, the conference was a fruitful exchange of views by experts in the field.
Whilst we all learned a great deal from each other, perhaps the most important
lesson which emerged was that there is no substitute for well-conducted clinical
medicine. Enthusiasm for new investigation should always be tempered by critical
assessment of results yet much new information is needed before we can approach the
problem of recognising coronary heart disease in the pre-clinical stage, let alone
preventing its subsequent ravages.

Supported by NHLBI Specialized Center of Research in Atherosclerosis, Grant HL-14138; NASA Office of Life Science Program, Medical Image Analysis Facility; and the Robert E. and May R. Wright Foundation

1. Professor of Medicine, Director - Cardiology, 2. Director, Biomedical Image Processing Laboratory, 3. Associate Professor of Medicine (Biomathematics)

NONINVASIVE IMAGING OF ATHEROSCLEROTIC LESIONS IN THE CAROTID ARTERIES OF PATIENTS

Bruce A. Kottke, Titus C. Evans, Jr. and James F. Greenleaf

Mayo Clinic and Foundation, Rochester, Minnesota, U.S.A.

Supported by Grant HV 42904 from the National Institutes of Health

INITIAL EVENTS IN ATHEROGENESIS

Colin J. Schwartz, M.D., F.R.A.C.P., F.R.C.Path.,[*] John B. Somer, Ph.D.[+] and Ross G. Gerrity, Ph.D.[*]

[*] The Department of Atherosclerosis and Thrombosis Research, The Cleveland Clinic Foundation, Ohio 44106, U.S.A.

[+] Department of Medicine, University of New South Wales, Prince Henry Hospital, Little Bay, N.S.W., 2036, Australia.

Supported in part by the Medical Research Council of Canada, The Ontario Heart Foundation, and the Cleveland Clinic Foundation

THE NON-INVASIVE DETECTION OF LATENT CORONARY ARTERY DISEASE

D. John Coltart and Patrick S. Robinson

The Department of Cardiology and Cardiac Research Laboratory, Rayne Institute, St. Thomas' Hospital, Medical School, London, S.E.1.

This study was supported by a research grant from Eli Lilly Ltd., United Kingdom

MAXIMAL EXERCISE TESTING - A PRELIMINARY REPORT OF THE SEATTLE HEART WATCH

Robert A. Bruce, M.D., Timothy DeRouen, Ph.D. and Barbara Blake, R.N.

Departments of Medicine and Biostatistics, RG-20, University of Washington, Seattle, Washington, 98195

This study has been supported by Research Contract HL 13517 and grant from the National Heart and Lung Institute, and grant MB 00184 from the Health Services Research Administration

RADIOACTIVE TRACERS IN THE EARLY RECOGNITION OF ISCHEMIC HEART DISEASE

Haile Selassie Lecture 1977

Bertram Pitt

Johns Hopkins Medical Institutions, Baltimore, Maryland, U.S.A.

SUDDEN DEATH

Desmond G. Julian, M.D., F.R.C.P.

British Heart Foundation Professor of Cardiology, University of Newcastle upon Tyne, Department of Cardiology, Newcastle General Hospital, Newcastle upon Tyne NE4 6BE

IMPLICATIONS OF REGIONAL CARDIAC MECHANICAL FUNCTION IN MYOCARDIAL ISCHEMIA AND INFARCTION - A Strategy for Presymptomatic Detection

H.J.C. Swan, M.D., James S. Forrester, M.D. and Ran Vas, Ph.D.

Department of Cardiology, Cedars-Sinai Medical Center, and the Department of Medicine, UCLA School of Medicine, Los Angeles, California

THE DETECTION OF INCOORDINATE LEFT VENTRICULAR CONTRACTION BY M-MODE ECHOCARDIOGRAPHY

D.G. Gibson

Brompton Hospital, London, SW3 6HP

MYOCARDIAL SCINTIGRAPHY AND RECONSTRUCTIVE TOMOGRAPHIC POSITRON IMAGING USING NITROGEN - 13 LABELLED AMMONIA

Leon Resnekov, Paul Harper, Frank Atkins and H. Karunaratne

Department of Medicine, Radiology and Surgery and the Franklin McLean Memorial Research Institute, University of Chicago Pritzker School of Medicine

Supported by USPHA Contract HV-81334 (Myocardial Infarction Research Unit), SCOR-Ischemic Heart Disease Grant HL 17648, USPHS Center for Imaging Research Grant GM-18940 and US Energy Research and Development Administration under ERDA Contract E (11-1)-69

CORONARY ARTERIOGRAPHY

P.S. Robinson and John Coltart

The Department of Cardiology and Cardiac Research Laboratory,
Rayne Institute, St. Thomas Hospital, Medical School, London S.E.1.

CORONARY VASOSPASM AS A CAUSE OF ANGINA PECTORIS

A. Maseri, M.D., A.L'Abbate, M.D., S. Chierchia, M.D., O. Parodi, M.D., M. Marzilli,
M.D., A.M. Ballestra, M.D., S. Severi, M.D., A. Distante, M.D. and A. Biagini, M.D.

Laboratorio di Fisiologia Clinica del C.N.R. and Istituto di Patologia Medica 1,
University of Pisa, Pisa, Italy